The National Pharmacy Technician Training Program

6th Edition
(2nd Printing)

Author
Kenneth W. Schafermeyer, R.Ph., Ph.D.

Managing Editor
Brandon M. Williams

The author has exercised care to assure that the information contained in this program is accurate and current at the time of writing. Because of the variable nature of pharmacy regulations and standards of practice, these organizations cannot be held liable for any activity resulting from the inappropriate use of information in this *Training Program*. This *Training Program* is not intended as legal advice; readers are urged to refer to the latest copy of their state's Drug Control Act and Regulations of their respective board of pharmacy.

Acknowledgements

The National Pharmacy Technician Training Program ("*Training Program*") was written by Kenneth W. Schafermeyer. Many people also contributed their expertise to the *Training Program* and their assistance is gratefully acknowledged. The following individuals contributed to the development of the *Training Program*:

- Kelly J. Burch, Pharm.D
- Rasma S. Chereson, R.Ph., Ph.D.
- Laura J. Cranston, R.Ph.
- Tony Dasher, Pharm.D.
- Deborah Faucette, R.Ph.
- Steven M. Gullette
- Eric H. Hobson, Ph.D.
- Deborah R. Holley, R.Ph
- Katherine Lenzi
- Justin Lusk, Pharm.D.
- Faith Nunn
- Jeffrey Martin, R.Ph.
- Rebecca M. Rabbitt, Pharm.D.
- Mayur V. Shah, Pharm.D.
- Robert Shapiro, R.Ph.
- C. Patrick Tharp, R.Ph., Ph.D.
- Brandon M. Williams, C.Ph.T.
- Tasha Williams, Pharm.D.
- Jeffrey Yue, Pharm.D.

Bulk discounts are available for this Training Program from the Institute for the Certification of Pharmacy Technicians (ICPT) for orders of 10 or more copies shipped together to the same address. Please contact ICPT for more information at 314-442-6775.

An Instructor's Manual is available to pharmacy technician instructors who have adopted ten or more copies of this *Training Program*. The Instructor's Manual includes learning objectives, key words, discussion questions and answers, suggested quiz problems and answers and in-class exercises. For more information, go to www.nationaltechexam.org or contact the ICPT office at 314-442-6775.

Forward

The important role that pharmacy technicians play in promoting medication safety continues to grow and gain more recognition by pharmacists, the media, and public policy officials. It is now common knowledge that well-trained pharmacy technicians not only make the pharmacy department more efficient, they also make it safer and more effective. The goal of *The National Pharmacy Technician Training Program* is to help pharmacy technicians prepare to serve in these expanded roles.

This new edition of the *Training Program* has been published to help pharmacy technicians and technician trainers keep up to date with the many changes occurring in health care and pharmacy. These changes include new drug products, new laws and regulations, changes in drug utilization patterns and advancements in technology.

This publication has gone through many significant changes during the 13 years it has been in print. *The National Pharmacy Technician Training Program* is currently published by the Institute for the Certification of Pharmacy Technicians (ICPT). The previous edition of the *Training Program* was published by Midwest Pharmaceutical Consultants, LLC and earlier editions were published by the Institute for the Advancement of Community Pharmacy under the title: *The Pharmacy Technician Training Program*. The first edition, published in 1995 by the National Association of Chain Drug Stores and the National Community Pharmacists Association, was known as the *Community Retail Pharmacy Technician Training Manual*. Since then, this publication has been updated, expanded and improved. Chapters were added to cover sterile products, unit dose and drug repackaging, federal privacy laws under HIPAA, basic medical terminology and basic anatomy and physiology. The managed care chapter has been revised numerous times to keep it up to date. Each new edition has reflected the most recent changes in federal laws and regulations. Additional self-assessment questions have been added. Chapters have been restructured and renumbered and the list of the top 200 drugs has been constantly updated.

The changes for the sixth edition continue our efforts to keep the *Training Program* up-to-date:

- A new chapter on over-the-counter (OTC) medications has been added, along with a useful table listing the most common OTC products by name, use and therapeutic class. Also included are tables outlining the uses for various vitamins, minerals and herbal products.
- An index has been added to help readers locate specific information.
- The chapters covering basic medical terminology and basic anatomy and physiology have been expanded to cover an additional organ system, more disease states and additional information on therapeutics.
- Useful information has been added to show how the suffix of a generic drug name can be used to help identify the therapeutic class of a given medication.
- The chapter on pharmacy calculations has been expanded to cover specific gravity, tonicity and milliequivalents.
- Information about dangerous medical abbreviations, verifying DEA numbers, the FDA *Orange Book* and useful FDA websites have been expanded.
- The top 200 list has been updated.

- All text and examples have been carefully reviewed and updated to keep them current.

Please Note: Please check the Manual Update Page on the ICPT website (http://www.nationaltechexam.org/tech_updates.shtml) for: (1) any corrections to this publication and (2) any new information that was not available for the *Training Program* before publication of this new edition. It is expected that there will soon be new information available about: (1) reimbursement for multiple-source products under Medicare and Medicaid, (2) tamper-resistant prescription pads and (3) changes in the expiration dating for repackaged products. This information will be posted as it becomes available.

In 2005, ICPT introduced The Exam for the Certification of Pharmacy Technicians (ExCPT)®, a nationally recognized and psychometrically sound pharmacy technician certification exam that has been declared by numerous state boards of pharmacy to be equivalent to the alternative exam in content and quality but less expensive and more convenient. (For more information about the ExCPT®, please visit the ICPT website at **www.nationaltechexam.org**.) Although this *Training Program* is not required for taking the ExCPT®, it is an excellent study guide. Items included on the ExCPT® are covered by this *Training Program*.

Kenneth W. Schafermeyer, R.Ph., Ph.D.
St. Louis, Missouri

Note: Unless noted otherwise, all photos used in this manual were purchased with a licensed royalty agreement from istock International, Inc.

The National Pharmacy Technician Training Program

TABLE OF CONTENTS

Exam for the Certification of Pharmacy Technicians (ExCPT®)

Purpose

The purpose of the Exam for the Certification of Pharmacy Technicians (ExCPT®) is to help ensure that a minimum knowledge base or competency is possessed by pharmacy technicians who assist pharmacists in the preparation of prescriptions. The ExCPT® is nationally recognized by the National Community Pharmacists Association and the National Association of Chain Drug Stores as a psychometrically sound pharmacy technician certification exam and is accredited by the National Commission for Certifying Agencies (NCCA).

Registration

Eligibility requirements. To be eligible to take the ExCPT®, a candidate must: (1) be at least 18 years of age, (2) have a high school diploma or GED and (3) have never been convicted of a felony. Candidates are encouraged to read the Candidates Guide posted on the ICPT website (www.nationaltechexam.org) for full information.

Contacting LaserGrade. The ExCPT® is offered over 310 days per year at over 300 PSI/ LaserGrade Testing Centers throughout the United States. Candidates may register by calling the LaserGrade toll-free number 1-800-211-2754 to arrange a test date, time and location. By providing a zip code, the candidate will be informed of the closest LaserGrade Testing Centers. Alternatively, these locations can be found on the Web at **www.lasergrade.com**. Exams can usually be taken within 24 to 48 hours of registration.

Information required. Candidates must give their full name, address, Social Security Number, telephone number, email address (if applicable) and demographic information such as date of birth, gender, employer, type of practice site, type of training, years of practice and hours worked per week. These data are used to analyze test results and produce reports. Date of birth also helps verify identification at the test center. Candidates should also indicate whether they qualify for special accommodations under the Americans with Disabilities Act.

Payment. The current price for the ExCPT® is posted on the ICPT website and is payable by credit card at the time the candidate registers. Candidates who do not have credit cards can send a check or money order. Employers may prepay for a specified number of candidates by making arrangements directly with LaserGrade. Registered candidates who need to change an exam time for any reason must contact the ICIP call center at least 24 hours in advance to reschedule or cancel an exam without penalty.

Preparing for the ExCPT®

Unless specified otherwise by an employer or by a given state board of pharmacy, candidates are not required to participate in a specific pharmacy technician training program in order to take the ExCPT®. *The National Pharmacy Technician Training Program*, which you are reading now, covers all content areas covered by the Exam and includes self-assessment questions and a competency assessment tool at the end of each module. The *Training Program* is also easy to incorporate into a new technician orientation program as well as on-going employee performance evaluation programs.

> **Note:** Be sure that you have a current copy of the *Training Program*. The sixth edition that you are reading now was published in the spring of 2008. The seventh edition is scheduled for spring 2009. To ensure that you have the latest information and are fully prepared for the ExCPT®, please check the ICPT website to make sure that you have the current edition. (www.nationaltechexam.org/shop_pttpm.shtml)

A description of the major areas covered on the ExCPT® is available on the ICPT website **www.nationaltechexam.org**. Candidates may also want to check their knowledge by using the Practice Exam that is available for a nominal fee on the ICPT website.

Taking the ExCPT®

The ExCPT® is a proctored, computer-based exam offered during business hours and some evenings and weekends at over 300 PSI/ LaserGrade Testing Centers throughout the United States. Candidate identification is verified at the LaserGrade Testing Center at the time of the test. The candidates have two hours to answer 110 multiple-choice questions. One question is presented on the screen at a time. Candidates may mark the answer or they can skip questions and come back later. Final answers are submitted when the candidate is finished and results are given immediately upon completion. A demonstration of the computer format used for exams administered by LaserGrade is shown on the LaserGrade website at **www.lasergrade.com**.

Scoring Exams and Reporting Results

Exam results for successful candidates. The ExCPT® is scored immediately and successful candidates are given an official report by LaserGrade indicating that they passed the ExCPT® immediately after completing the exam. Candidates may use this report to provide evidence to employers or regulatory boards that they passed the Exam and are a certified pharmacy technician.

Exam results for unsuccessful candidates. The purpose of the exam is to provide summative assessment (i.e., to determine whether an individual has achieved a certain level of competency). It is not designed for formative assessment (i.e., to give the candidate feedback). ICPT does, however, provide diagnostic reports to help unsuccessful candidates focus their study time so they can successfully retake the exam. This diagnostic report will indicate how the candidate performed on each of nine major sections of the exam. A description of the specific content from each of these sections of the exam can be found on the ICPT website. Candidates can also get some feedback by taking the Practice Exam offered on the ICPT website.

Recognition of certification. Pharmacy technicians who successfully pass the ExCPT® are considered Certified Pharmacy Technicians and may use the designation "CPhT" after their name. A certificate suitable for framing and a wallet identification card are sent to CPhTs within a few weeks.

Reexamination. Candidates who do not pass the ExCPT® will be allowed to retake the exam after four weeks. Since there are multiple versions of the ExCPT®, candidates who take retake the exam will receive a different, but equivalent, set of questions.

Recertification

Application. Certification is valid for two years and expires on the date listed on the official certificate. During the two-year period prior to recertification, certified pharmacy technicians must participate in at least 20 hours of continuing education (CE), including at least one hour of pharmacy law. To recertify, technicians must use the ICPT recertification application form and may file either online or by regular mail. Complete instructions are provided with the form. Address changes should be sent to the Institute so that we may send a recertification application approximately 60 days prior to the expiration date. Technicians will be allowed to recertify up to 90 days after expiration of their certification but cannot include CE credit earned during this grace period. After this 90-day period, there will be a late fee.

Continuing education. To be approved, CE credit must be related to pharmacy technician practice. Acceptable topics include, but are not limited to: drug distribution, inventory control, managed health care, drug products, therapeutic issues, patient interaction, communication and interpersonal skills, pharmacy operations, prescription compounding, calculations, pharmacy law, preparation of sterile products and drug repackaging.

Certificates of participation must be obtained for each CE program. This certificate must include the name of the participant, the title of the program, date of the program, number of contact hours, the name of the sponsor and the signature of the person responsible for the program.

CE programs offered by national and state pharmacy associations and pharmacy technician associations will generally be acceptable if related to pharmacy technician practice. Applicable college courses with a grade of "C" or better will also be eligible for CE credit at the rate of 15 CE hours for each 3 credit-hour course offered on a semester basis (i.e., three hours per week for 15 weeks). Courses offered on a quarter basis will be credited for 15 hours for a 4 credit-hour course (i.e., four hours per week for approximately 11 weeks). The maximum number of CE credits earned through college courses during a two-year period is 15.

Ongoing Training and Competency
Assessment Plan

HOW TO USE THIS TRAINING PROGRAM

This *Training Program* is designed to be used by community pharmacy technician trainees and pharmacists as a training aid. It is only through the close interaction of technician trainees and pharmacists that patients will receive a high level of quality care and services. Therefore, directions are given to both parties about how they might make the most of this *Training Program.*

Notes to Pharmacy Technician Trainees

You are undertaking a period of intense activity as you work to learn the information and master all of the skills you will need to be a competent pharmacy technician. While there is a large amount of material presented here, rest assured that you can learn it. What you need is a strategy for studying this material. Good students know a few proven strategies that can help them learn faster. Here are a few strategies to help you study:

- **Read the chapters one at a time.** While it is tempting to flip through books, it is not very efficient. Most books are designed to be used in a set sequence. This *Training Program* is no exception.

  The chapters in this *Training Program* build on each other. This means that information presented in Chapter I, for instance, lays the base for information that you will encounter as you read Chapter II and even Chapter VIII.

- **Take notes; ask yourself questions.** As you read, you will undoubtedly see information that you know is so important that you must not forget it. When this happens, make a note of it.

- **Ask your trainer questions.** There will be much in the following pages that seem difficult at first. For instance, all the regulations about what you may and may not do as a technician may seem extreme. However, you are surrounded by people who can help you understand. And they will help, if you ask them to help you. Remember that there are no dumb questions when patients' good health is at stake. A good practice to follow is, "If in doubt, ask." It's a good idea to set aside a few minutes at the beginning or end of a shift to ask questions and discuss issues that may seem confusing.

- **Use the learning objectives, sample questions and assessment statements.** The learning objectives at the beginning of each chapter summarize the information and skills that each chapter covers. The learning objectives are designed to help you focus on the main points so that you can get the most out of each chapter.

  At the end of each chapter are sample questions which you can use to test your knowledge and review the information you have read. The assessment statements at the end of each chapter serve this same purpose but can also assist you and your trainer to keep track of the progress you make and to focus on those areas where you need to learn more. Make a note of those areas that you have not yet mastered and use them to help set goals for future improvement.

- **Refer to your pharmacy's Policy and Procedure Manual.** The information in the following pages is designed to reflect how a typical pharmacy operates. Since individual pharmacies will differ, there may be areas where the policies and procedures followed in your pharmacy will be a bit different. In cases such as this, always follow your pharmacy's rules. This is why we recommend that you also review your pharmacy's Policy and Procedure Manual during the training process.

- **Use the glossary.** At the end of this *Training Program* is a glossary that defines many of the terms which you will need to know. It's a good idea to refer to the glossary whenever you encounter an unfamiliar term and when you want to check your knowledge.

- **Review this information.** Hang on to this *Training Program*. Even after you complete you pharmacy technician training, there will be times when you need to brush up on the information. Early on, you may need to review the *Training Program* on a regular basis.

Notes to Trainers

As noted in the previous section, your technician trainee is going through a demanding training process. As with every period when we are asked to learn large amounts of new information, questions can arise. The technician trainee likely will have many questions that need answers. Because the technician is working in your store, those answers need to be specific. Therefore, you need to be the one to supply them.

With this in mind, we offer you the following advice about using this *Training Program*.

- **Read the Training Program.** This document is designed as a learning aid and is intended to be used in sequence, from front to back. As such, you need to know exactly what topics are covered and in what order so that you can maximize learning.

- **Make notes of differences.** Some of the information contained in the following pages will not correlate exactly to the policies and procedures followed in your pharmacy. This document is written for a general audience; therefore, you will need to inform your technician trainees where your policies and procedures may differ from what is presented in this *Training Program*.

We suggest that you supplement this *Training Program* with pages that explain the particular rules and regulations of your state. You may want to bring the appropriate information to the attention of your trainees and supplement it with your own instructions when necessary.

- **Anticipate questions.** Technician trainees typically have many questions, usually the same questions. Because of the redundant nature of many of these questions, we suggest that you consider adding a list of common questions and detailed answers and explanations to each chapter. To stimulate thinking and discussion, we have added a few practice problems at the end of each chapter. You may also want to review these in case trainees ask for explanations.

- **Conduct assessments.** If this *Training Program* does its intended job, your technician trainees should be better prepared to function as productive pharmacy technicians. They will be able to meet your high expectations, however, only if you work with them. A collaborative effort during the learning process is essential to continued development of their knowledge and abilities, especially when you assess their progress along the way.

One way to assess technician trainees' knowledge is to verify their understanding of the terminology defined in the Glossary at the end of this *Training Program*. Another suggestion is to use the assessments at the end of each chapter which are designed to allow both you and the technician trainee to be able to openly assess and discuss the level of development attained in specific areas. We suggest that they be used not only as assessments of material mastered, but as opportunities for setting goals for future improvement and discussing challenges that lie ahead.

An Instructor's Manual is available to pharmacy technician instructors who have adopted ten or more copies of this *Training Program*. The Instructor's Manual includes learning objectives, key words, discussion questions and answers, suggested quiz problems and answers and in-class exercises. For more information, go to www.nationaltechexam.org or contact the ICPT office at 314-442-6775.

Chapter I

Basic Overview

EDUCATIONAL OBJECTIVES

After studying the material in this chapter, the technician trainee should be able to:

- Describe the functions a technician may perform
- Describe the functions a technician may not perform
- Understand the importance of confidentiality to the practice of pharmacy
- Understand the general layout of the pharmacy department
- Describe the federal and state agencies and regulations affecting pharmacy
- Describe the role of the state board of pharmacy

JOB OVERVIEW

In choosing to become a pharmacy technician, you have selected a challenging and rewarding occupation. You will become an important member of the pharmacy's health care team. Technicians increase the pharmacy's efficiency by helping pharmacists prepare prescriptions. This, in turn, allows pharmacists to spend more time providing professional services such as:

- Counseling patients (i.e., making sure patients know how to take their medications)
- Monitoring therapy (i.e., making sure patients are taking their medications according to the prescriber's directions)
- Performing interventions (i.e., working with prescribers to improve drug therapy)

Your work is challenging because of its variety. The work involves two general types of activities: processing prescriptions and maintaining the pharmacy department.

In the first role, you may:
- Receive refill requests from patients over the phone
- Obtain patient health information
- Receive refill authorizations from nurses or physicians over the phone
- Enter data in the computer
- Retrieve medications from shelves
- Print prescription labels
- Prepare medications for a pharmacist to check
- Submit insurance billing/enter insurance information into the computer

In the second role, you may:
- Order medications
- Stock the pharmacy department
- Keep accurate records for the pharmacy department
- Help patients locate over-the-counter (OTC) medications (i.e., medications that are available without a prescription)

Being a pharmacy technician involves reacting to what is happening around you and anticipating the needs of both patients and pharmacists.

Your work also requires responsibility. You will always work under the supervision of one or more pharmacists who will assign you responsibilities and tasks described in this *Training Program*. If your state permits pharmacy technicians to prepare prescriptions, pharmacists will always check your work before medications are given to patients or their caregivers.

Your days will be fast-paced, interesting, and challenging. If you are a person who takes initiative, thrives on variety and responsibility, and enjoys being a part of a team, you will find your work rewarding.

As an important part of the pharmacy team, you will have to anticipate pharmacists' and patients' needs. In meeting these needs, however, it is extremely important that you follow the pharmacy's policies and procedures and pharmacists' instructions precisely. You must follow these guidelines for three crucial reasons:

1. Anything you do shapes the image of the pharmacy in patients' eyes.
2. Pharmacists are legally and professionally responsible for your actions.
3. Mistakes can seriously affect patients' health.

Technician Duties

Depending on your state's laws and your pharmacy department's policies and procedures, your responsibilities may include those listed in the following sample job description.

SAMPLE JOB DESCRIPTION

Title: Pharmacy Technician

Reports to: Pharmacist(s) on duty

General Responsibilities: To assist pharmacists in processing prescriptions and maintaining the pharmacy department.

Specific Responsibilities:
- Answer telephone and handle questions that do not require a pharmacist's expertise or judgment.
- Receive written prescriptions or telephoned refill requests.
- Gather information needed to prepare prescriptions.
- Record information needed before prescriptions can be dispensed.
- Store written prescription forms after prescriptions are dispensed.
- Enter data into the computer.
- Notify pharmacists of patient or prescriber questions and medication warnings or interactions.
- Help pharmacists prepare prescriptions by counting or pouring medications, labeling containers, and pricing prescriptions.
- Keep pharmacy department supplies (e.g., bottles, bags, receipts, staples, etc.) well-stocked.
- Place completed prescriptions in the pick-up area.
- Order and check-in the pharmacy department shelves with medications when they arrive from suppliers.
- Prepare insurance claims and verify payments.
- Help patients find over-the-counter medications.
- Stock over-the-counter departments.
- Ring purchases on cash registers and record them in logs when necessary.
- Perform housekeeping duties within the pharmacy department.

Internal Contacts: Works closely with pharmacists. Also works with cashiers, clerks and other store personnel.

External Contacts: Works with patients, patients' caregivers, prescribers and their office personnel and with suppliers to the pharmacy.

Duties Pharmacy Technicians Cannot Perform

Certain duties cannot be assigned to you because they can only be performed by pharmacists. These restrictions are regulated at state and federal levels and you must follow them closely.

- Only pharmacists can receive oral prescriptions from prescribers or prescribers' authorized designees. (This refers primarily to new telephone prescriptions and refill authorizations where there are changes to the prescriptions.)
- Only pharmacists can consult with prescribers or prescribers' designees about patients' prescriptions.
- Only pharmacists can provide confidential patient information to other health professionals or insurance companies.
- Only pharmacists can check medications before dispensing them to patients. (In states where technicians can prepare or package prescriptions, they do so under the direct supervision of a pharmacist.)
- Only pharmacists can consult with patients about prescribed medication use and other health issues.
- Only pharmacists can recommend over-the-counter medications.

Confidentiality

Pharmacists are among the most trusted professional people. Preserving patient confidentiality is important to maintaining this trust. **It is crucial that you keep personal or health information about patients strictly confidential at all times.** Discussing a patient's health information with **anyone** other than the patient, the patient's caregiver, or the pharmacists you work with is a serious violation of ethics and could expose the pharmacy to a law suit. It is imperative that pharmacy technicians know the patient confidentiality requirements of the Health Insurance Portability and Accountability Act (HIPAA) that went into effect in April 2003. These requirements are discussed later in this *Training Program.*

DEPARTMENT LAYOUT

The pharmacy department, whether in a community or hospital setting, is managed for efficiency. Equipment, products, and work stations are located for convenience, accuracy, and speed. Depending upon how many prescriptions your pharmacy department dispenses, you may have several types of staff members attending to duties but managing not to crowd each other in the process.

The staff may include pharmacy clerks, pharmacy technicians, pharmacy interns, and pharmacists. To maximize function and workflow, the pharmacy department is divided into two major areas: the medication storage area and the dispensing work area.

Medication Storage Area

Medication bays. The medication storage areas are usually U-shaped shelving units on which medications are kept. These "bays," as they are known, are arranged so you or a pharmacist can reach more medications with fewer steps, thus reducing the time needed to fill prescriptions. The two most common methods of arranging storage bays are described below. These arrangements can be found in various combinations among pharmacy departments.

- **Arranged alphabetically by brand name.** Medications may simply be arranged from A to Z according to brand name. Generic equivalents are usually placed immediately beside their brands although some pharmacy departments also alphabetize the generics.

- **Arranged by package size or dosage form.** Arranging oversized packages (e.g., one-gallon bottles) or undersized packages (e.g., eye drops) on their own shelves saves space. Some pharmacies separate some dosage forms (e.g., topical creams and ointments) from other stock and alphabetize them by brand name.

Speed shelf. Located in the dispensing area, this shelf holds medications prescribed most often. This area is sometimes called the "fast-mover section." These medications are dispensed repeatedly during the day; therefore, the product packages (i.e., stock bottles) are usually kept nearby for easy access. Some pharmacy departments locate speed shelves above their work counter where prescriptions are filled. Other pharmacy departments use the narrow shelving units at the ends of the U-shaped medication bays.

Refrigerator. The refrigerator contains medications, such as insulin and liquid antibiotics, that must be kept cool until use. Food should not be stored in the same refrigerator with medications.

Work Areas

Smooth, efficient work flow helps pharmacists dispense prescriptions more quickly with a minimum of errors. Work generally flows in one direction along the prescription counter; each part of the counter has its own specific function. This section describes these work areas and typical work flow behind prescription counters.

In-window. The counter area where you greet patients and obtain patient information about new prescriptions and refills is sometimes called the "In-window." Because this area creates the patient's first impression of the pharmacy department, keep it clean and uncluttered. It should be free of signs, displays, or supplies that interfere with patient service.

Out-window. The counter area where pharmacists counsel patients and you or members of the staff complete the sales transaction is sometimes called the "Out-window." Also keep this area uncluttered since patients need room to sign various forms and write checks. Some pharmacy departments have only one counter or window which they use as both an in-and out-window; others have separate counseling areas with more privacy to discuss confidential matters.

The data-entry area is the work station where the computer is located. Sometimes this area is next to the in-window. Here you enter information into patient profiles. Prescription labels are prepared on a printer located in the dispensing area (which is described below). The data-entry area has three functional components whose specific arrangements in the pharmacy department may vary.

- **The "to-be-entered" section,** typically located next to the computer, holds prescription forms until they are keyed into the computer. To reduce patient waiting time, prescription forms for patients who are waiting are placed ahead of prescription forms for patients who will return later to pick up their prescriptions.

- **The "to-be-filled" section,** usually a rack or filing system, is organized by pick-up times. Prescriptions are prepared by working your way through this file according to pick-up times. The filing system organizes your work and it helps assure that prescriptions are ready when patients expect them to be.

- **The "staging" section** is the counter space next to, or near, the dispensing area. The label, original prescription order, and stock bottles of medications to dispense are placed in this staging area.

The dispensing area is that part of the counter space where you count, pour and package medications. Keep this area well-organized and clutter free. Only equipment needed to dispense medication should be allowed in the area. Mix-ups here are serious.

- **Counting equipment,** counting trays and automatic pill counters are located here. This equipment, described later in this *Training Program,* varies among pharmacies.

- **A distilled water dispenser** is usually located near the work area. Distilled water is added to pre-measured powders to create solutions or suspensions. These "reconstitutables," usually antibiotics, have short shelf-lives after water is added. They often require refrigeration.

- **Auxiliary labels** provide written reminders to patients such as: "Take all medication," "Do not mix with alcohol," or "Take with food or milk." They come in rolls, much like postage stamps, and are kept in a dispenser in the work area.

- **A calculator** may be kept on hand to compute dosage amounts.

- **Prescription containers** are usually stored within easy reach under the prescription counter. Less frequently used containers are often stored nearby.

Other areas where you will work are storage areas, administrative offices, clean rooms, and the front of the store. Specifically, these areas include:

- **The pick-up area** is a group of bins or baskets where finished prescriptions await pick up. Prescriptions are usually stored in the bins alphabetically by patients' last names.

- **The administration area** is used to complete paperwork and to check in orders from suppliers.

- **The over-the-counter (OTC) area** contains nonprescription medications. It is typically located close to the prescription department to make it easy for pharmacists to recommend specific products or answer questions about OTC products.

- **The clean room** is a controlled environment for compounding sterile products in hospitals and other pharmacies that provide home infusion services. Laminar flow hoods (which are described in the chapter on Sterile Product Compounding) are located in this area.

LAWS AFFECTING PRESCRIPTION DISPENSING

Because pharmacists control the use of medications that are potentially dangerous or have high potential for abuse, pharmacy is one of the most highly-regulated professions in America. Numerous laws affecting pharmacy are enforced by both federal and state governments. When both the federal and state government addresses a particular situation, the stricter law applies. Listed below are examples of some areas of pharmacy practice that federal and state governments regulate:

Approval of Medications for Use in the United States

The Food and Drug Administration (FDA) is the federal agency that supervises the development, testing, purity, safety, and effectiveness of prescription and OTC medications. The FDA must approve medications before they can be sold in the United States. The FDA also regulates the advertising of prescription medications and the labeling of prescription and OTC medications.

Controlled Substances

Controlled substances are medications with significant potential for abuse (e.g., narcotics, amphetamines, and barbiturates). The Comprehensive Drug Abuse Prevention and Control Act of 1970 — more commonly referred to as the Controlled Substance Act (CSA) regulates manufacturing, distribution, prescribing, and dispensing of controlled substances through the Drug Enforcement Administration (DEA). Prescribers are assigned DEA numbers which authorize them to prescribe controlled substances. Always check for the presence of DEA numbers on prescriptions written for controlled substances. Controlled substances are discussed in more detail in Chapter III.

Child-Resistant Containers

The Consumer Product Safety Commission (CPSC) oversees the 1970 Poison Prevention Packaging Act. The CPSC requires most prescriptions for oral use to be dispensed in child-resistant containers unless patients or prescribers request otherwise.

Note: There is an important exception to this rule. Nitroglycerin sublingual tablets must be dispensed in the original, unopened container, labeled with the following statement directed to the patient: "Warning: to prevent loss of potency, keep these tablets in the original container or in a supplemental Nitroglycerin container specifically labeled as being suitable for Nitroglycerin Tablets. Close tightly immediately after each use."

Patient Counseling

The Omnibus Budget Reconciliation Act of 1990 (OBRA '90) is a federal law that increases pharmacists' professional responsibilities in two ways:

1. OBRA '90 requires pharmacists to keep records (i.e., patient profiles) of all medications used by Medicaid patients. These patient records help reduce the incidence of medication therapy problems due to drug duplication, allergies, drug interactions, drug side effects, and patients' misuse or abuse of prescribed medications.

2. OBRA '90 requires pharmacists to offer to counsel all Medicaid patients about the proper use of their medications.

The requirements of OBRA '90 are now interpreted to include all patients — not just those covered by Medicaid. Every patient profile must undergo prospective (prior to dispensing) and retrospective (periodic) drug utilization reviews (DUR). These two requirements have helped expand the use of pharmacy technicians as a way to allow pharmacists more time to counsel patients and perform other professional services. While only pharmacists can counsel patients, technicians can gather information for patient records and become more involved in dispensing activities.

State Boards of Pharmacy

State boards of pharmacy license all pharmacists and pharmacy departments within their state. Pharmacy boards regulate the operation of pharmacy departments, and the practice of pharmacy by pharmacists as well as the performance of technical functions by pharmacy technicians. Each board is responsible for protecting its citizens' health and welfare, with regard to pharmacy services.

Boards employ inspectors and/or investigators to inspect pharmacies for compliance with state pharmacy laws and regulations. Inspectors conduct regular inspections of licensed pharmacy departments. State pharmacy boards can revoke, suspend, or place on probation licenses of those who are found guilty, after due process, of violating laws or regulations.

Your state's board of pharmacy regulates many tasks you perform as a technician (e.g., generic substitution, licensing requirements, computer records, labeling, etc.). *It is important that you check with the pharmacist about your state's requirements on these issues.*

Joint Commission on Accreditation of Healthcare Organizations (JCAHO)

JCAHO is an organization that sets forth standards for organizations such as hospitals. Hospitals that meet these standards become accredited. To see if your hospital or organization is accredited, please visit the following site: http://www.qualitycheck.org

Pharmacy Security

Because of the presence of medications in the pharmacy department, the staff must take precautions to keep the area secure. Here are some general guidelines about how to maintain security. The pharmacist must:

- Keep the pharmacy department's entrance and exit doors closed and not allow sales representatives and unauthorized people to enter.

- Not allow store personnel to enter the pharmacy department unless they are scheduled to work in that area at that specific time.

- Keep the pharmacy department locked and inaccessible whenever a pharmacist is not on duty.

PHARMACY DEPARTMENT REFERENCE SOURCES

It is essential for every pharmacy department to have reference sources on hand to verify medication information. State boards of pharmacy may require your pharmacy department to keep certain references on hand at all times. Pharmacy literature is divided into three types: primary, secondary and tertiary. Primary literature includes original reports of clinical trials published in professional journals; secondary literature consists of reference works and search engines; tertiary literature encompasses text books, based on primary literature. Following is a short description of some pharmacy reference resources.

Package Inserts

Complete labeling and dispensing information must accompany all prescription medications from the manufacturer. Because prescription medications require more information than can be included on the label, a detailed package insert is either attached to the container itself or is placed inside the package. This information is written for pharmacists and prescribers, and is usually not intended to be given to patients. Package inserts include:

- **Product description.** The active ingredients, chemical name and formula, and characteristics of the product.

- **Indications for use.** A description of conditions the medication may be used to treat.

- **Contraindications.** Circumstances under which the medication should not be used.

- **Warnings.** Descriptions of extreme side effects, given certain conditions and special circumstances.

- **Precautions.** Information similar to warnings, but not as severe. The following issues are covered by precautions:

  1. Describes side effects that might be seen or expected but are not usually life-threatening.

  2. Lists conditions or diseases for which special care must be taken when prescribing the product.

  3. Notes interactions with other medications.

  4. Warns against possible tissue changes, impairment of fertility, or possible birth defects in pregnant or nursing women.

- **Adverse reactions.** Describes known side-effects and laboratory tests with which this medication may interfere; may also include statistics describing the percentage of the population that experiences these side-effects.

- **Dosage and administration.** Discusses correct doses for conditions the medication may be used to treat and for various other conditions or circumstances, including administration to children or elderly patients or patients with reduced liver or kidney function.

Patient Package Insert

Much of the same information contained in the package insert will be repeated in the patient package insert provided by the manufacturer, only in a form that is easier for non-medical persons to understand. Patient package inserts are required to accompany some medications, such as oral contraceptives, Accutane®, Premarin®, and metered-dose inhalers.

United States Pharmacopeia-National Formulary (USP-NF)

The *USP-NF* defines the standards for medications. The publication contains official titles of medications, standards for strength, purity, packaging and labeling, procedures for proper handling and storage, and formulas for manufacture or preparation.

United States Pharmacopeia Drug Information (USP-DI)

This book is available in two versions: patient and professional.

- *USP-DI Advice for the Patient* is a reference book which contains easy-to-understand Information about prescription medications for the non-medical person: how to take medications, what they will do, and their side effects. Many pharmacists keep the patient version of the USP-DI at the checkout counter so patients can learn about their medications. Some pharmacy departments will photocopy appropriate pages for their patients to take home.

- *USP-DI for the Health Care Professional* has more detailed, technical information. It is designed to be used by a pharmacist or other medical personnel. It contains information similar to *Drug Facts and Comparisons,* such as dispensing and prescribing information, interactions, allergies, warnings, and side effects.

Drug Facts and Comparisons (DFC)

This book (also available as a computer software program) is an encyclopedia of medications that contains many facts about product groups and individual products and makes comparisons among them. It contains complete dispensing and prescribing information, interactions, allergies, warnings, indications for use, and side effects. It also lists whether products are prescription or non-prescription medications. If a medication is a controlled substance, *Drug Facts and Comparisons* will indicate its schedule. It also contains relative price comparisons for drug products.

American Hospital Formulary Services Drug Information (AHFS-DI)

The *AHFS-DI* is a cornerstone in pharmacy practice and medicine due to the critically evaluated, evidenced-based and comparative collection of drug monographs on practically every single-drug entity available in the U.S. Originally developed by the American Society of Hospital Pharmacists to assist each hospital's pharmacy-and-therapeutics committee in selecting the most cost-effective treatments for various health conditions, it has become a widely-used source of complete drug information including description, usage, dosage and administration, cautions, drug interactions, chemistry and stability, and toxicity. The information is submitted by members of the National Institutes of Health, the Centers for Disease Control and Prevention, and other health-care organizations.

Physicians' Desk Reference (PDR)

The *PDR* is a listing of over 4,000 current brand and generic drugs with descriptions and information on their usage, warnings, drug interactions, category and more than 2,000 full-size, color photos. It is an annually updated reference and is considered the standard prescription drug information source by physicians.

Approved Drug Products with Therapeutic Equivalence Evaluations

Commonly called the "Orange Book," FDA's *Approved Drugs Products with Therapeutic Equivalent Evaluations* is a list of all FDA-approved prescription and over-the-counter drug products rated for safety and effectiveness, as well as bioequivalence. It is the basis for generic product selection by pharmacists.

Handbook on Injectable Drugs

The *Handbook on Injectable Drugs* is a key reference used in hospital and home-infusion settings. The information provided is based on the results of primary research of parenteral drug stability and compatibility. This book discusses storage requirements and general stability information, including pH, freezing, exposure to light, and repackaging information. It also provides key product data including common sizes, strengths, volumes, and dosage forms.

Handbook of Nonprescription Drugs

The *Handbook of Nonprescription Drugs* is the gold-standard on self-care and over-the-counter medications. This handbook is not only a textbook for many pharmacy students; it is an essential reference in any community pharmacy. It lists the safety and effectiveness of non-prescription medications, herbal remedies, homeopathic products, nutritional supplements, and home medical equipment. It features brief descriptions of the drug classes, usage, dosing and administration, case studies and patient counseling suggestions.

Useful FDA Websites[1]

Professional Development
> *CDERLearn* – Offers free online continuing education seminars on topics such as the brand- and generic-name approval process. www.fda.gov/cder/learn/CDERLearn

Pharmacy Practice
> *Drugs@FDA* – Catalog of approved prescription, over-the-counter, and discontinued drugs. Includes therapeutic equivalents, labels, and drug review packages. http://www.accessdata.fda.gov/scripts/cder/drugsatfda/

> *Drug Information Pathfinder* – Includes links to information on drug approvals, drug shortages, and recalls. www.fda.gov/cder/Offices/DDI/pathfinder.htm

> *New Requirements for Prescribing Information*
> www.fda.gov/cder/regulatory/physLabel

> *Eliminate Ambiguous Medical Abbreviations* – The Institute for Safe Medical Practices (ISMP) educates how to promote safe practices by eliminating dangerous abbreviations. www.fda.gov/cder/drug/MedErrors/#abbreviations

Patient Information
> *Medication Guides* – FDA-approved medication guide printouts available. http://www.fda.gov/cder/Offices/ODS/medication_guides.htm

> *Consumer Education: What you Need to Use Medications Safely*
> www.fda.gov/usemedicinesafely

Medication Safety
> *FDA's Drug Safety Initiative* – Drug-specific safety information for patients and health personnel. www.fda.gov/cder/drug/DrugSafety/DrugIndex.htm

> *Medwatch* – A site for consumers and health care personnel to report adverse events and medical product problems. www.fda.gov/medwatch

Most Up-to-Date Information
> *FDA's E-mail Newsletters* – Stay current on the latest information by choosing from more than 30 free FDA newsletters sent via email. www.fda.gov/emaillist.html

---

[1] The website links above may expire if the FDA makes changes to its website. If a website link does not work, you can still access the referenced information by visiting www.FDA.gov.

SELF-ASSESSMENT QUESTIONS CHAPTER I

1. According to the *Training Program,* functions that technicians are generally allowed to perform include:
   a. Receive oral prescriptions from prescribers.
   b. Tell patients how to use their medication.
   c. Receive refill request from patients over the telephone.
   d. Recommend over-the-counter medications.

2. The agency that supervises the development, testing, purity, safety and effectiveness of prescription and over-the-counter medications is known as the:
   a. Board of Pharmacy.
   b. Consumer Product Safety Commission (CPSC).
   c. Federal Trade Commission (FTC).
   d. Drug Enforcement Agency (DEA).
   e. Food and Drug Administration (FDA).

3. Which of the following is true regarding pharmacy department security?
   a. All entrance and exit doors to the pharmacy department must be closed.
   b. Schedule II, III and IV medications must be stored in a safe or locked in a secure cabinet.
   c. Employees from other parts of the store and sales representatives are allowed in the prescription department as long as the pharmacy is not too busy.
   d. The pharmacy department's hours must always be the same as the hours for the rest of the store.

4. State boards of pharmacy:
   a. Regulate prices of prescription drugs.
   b. Supervise the development, testing, purity, safety, and effectiveness of prescription and OTC medications.
   c. Represent the interest of pharmacists to the state legislature and other state agencies.
   d. Regulate the manufacturing of controlled substances.
   e. Are responsible for protecting their citizens' health and welfare with regard to pharmacy services.

5. Which of the following publications is the official information on generic equivalence?
   a. *USP-NF.*
   b. *USP-DI.*
   c. *PDR.*
   d. *DFC.*
   e. *Orange Book.*

Answers: 1) c   2) e   3) a   4) e   5) e

PHARMACY TECHNICIAN COMPETENCY ASSESSMENT
CHAPTER I

Description of Ability or Skill	Initials		Training Completed	
	Tech	R.Ph.	Date	Remarks
The technician trainee knows what functions a technician may perform and has cited such examples.				
The technician trainee knows the functions a technician may not perform and has cited such examples.				
The technician trainee understands and can explain what confidentiality is and why it is important to the practice of pharmacy.				
The technician trainee is familiar with the general layout of the pharmacy department and can locate specific areas and describe the functions carried out there.				
The technician trainee has demonstrated knowledge of federal and state agencies and regulations affecting pharmacy.				
The technician trainee can explain the role of the state board of pharmacy.				

Chapter II
Prescription Medications - General

EDUCATIONAL OBJECTIVES

After studying the material in this chapter, the technician trainee should be able to:

- Describe the characteristics of the four major categories of dosage forms
- Describe the characteristics of prescription containers and closures
- Locate prescription containers and closures in the pharmacy department
- Understand the state's rules and the pharmacy's policies regarding generic substitution
- Identify the information found on stock bottle labels
- Describe appropriate strategies for avoiding mix-ups among easily-confused products

DOSAGE FORMS

Medications often consist of very small quantities of chemicals known as "active ingredients" combined with inactive ingredients to make convenient dosage forms. Dosage forms are designed to help patients take medications by improving taste, appearance, stability, availability, and absorption. Some medications are prepared in more than one dosage form. You should always be sure that dosage forms dispensed are the same as those prescribed.

Oral Solid Dosage Forms

Capsules are small, oblong gelatin "containers" filled with medication. Some capsule designs are trademarked by manufacturers and may have special names. Many patients prefer capsules over tablets; capsules are easier to swallow because of their shape and because their gelatin exteriors become slippery when patients take them with water.

Tablets are solid dosage forms that vary greatly in shape, size, weight, and many other properties. Most tablets are swallowed whole with water and later break apart and dissolve in the digestive tract. Some tablets are scored with a groove that allows the tablet to be broken easily so patients can take a fraction of the dose.

There are several types of tablets including:

- **Buccal tablets** are placed in the buccal pouch (i.e., the area between the cheek and gums). From there, active ingredients are absorbed directly into the blood stream without passing through the digestive tract. Buccal tablets dissolve slowly.

- **Sublingual tablets** are placed under the tongue. They dissolve rapidly and are absorbed directly into the blood stream without passing through the digestive tract.

- **Chewable tablets** are intended to be chewed before swallowing. Most tablets should not be chewed unless specifically indicated as "chewable."

- **Effervescent tablets** contain mixtures of acids and sodium bicarbonate plus active ingredients. These "bubbling" tablets release carbon dioxide and dissolve rapidly in water. Effervescent tablets should not be chewed or swallowed, but always dissolved in a glass of water first which patients then drink.

- **Enteric-coated tablets** are coated to prevent them from dissolving in the stomach where they may be neutralized or rendered inactive by stomach acids; they dissolve in the intestine instead.

- **Troches and lozenges** are held in the mouth while they dissolve. These tablets keep the medication in contact with the mouth and throat for an extended period of time.

Pills were originally made from powdered raw materials such as leaves, roots, or ground animal glands. The powdered material was mixed with a sticky liquid, such as sugar syrup, formed into a pencil-shaped rod, and cut into equal parts. Each subdivision was then rolled into a round mass called a pill.

People often refer to any solid, oral, dosage forms as "Pills." However, very few official preparations are known as "Pills." When referring to oral contraceptives or any other solid-oral dosage form, it is more professional to call them "Tablets" or "capsules," whichever is appropriate.

Controlled-release products release medication over extended time periods to avoid high concentrations in the digestive tract or to provide longer durations of action than are available through conventional dosage forms. Tablets, capsules, or in some cases, medication particles themselves are specially coated to release portions of the medication in the body at specific times. These dosage forms usually contain two to four times the regular dose of medication which is released in the body over a period of eight to 24 hours.

Many medications are supplied in both immediate-release and controlled-release forms; sometimes their strengths are identical, as shown in the following examples:

Immediate-Release	*Controlled-Release*
Isordil® 40 mg tabs	Isordil® **Tembids** 40 mg caps
Inderal® 60 mg tabs	Inderal® **LA** 60 mg caps

You must know these products so you do not mistake one for another. Confusing one dosage form for another could cause under or overdoses and harm patients.

Controlled-release products are identified by their manufacturers in various ways. For example:

- **LA** (Long Acting)
- **SA** (Sustained Action)
- **SR** (Sustained Release)
- **CR** (Controlled Release)
- **XR/XL** (Extended Release)
- **TR** (Timed Release)

Oral Liquid Dosage Forms

You will dispense many liquid formulations. Most oral liquid medications are dissolved or suspended in a liquid—usually water, but sometimes alcohol or another suitable solvent. Most orally-ingested liquids also contain sugar and flavoring agents to improve taste.

Solutions are preparations in which the solid ingredients of medications are dissolved in a liquid (usually water). Solutions may have color but are usually clear—you can see through them.

Suspensions are substances in which medication particles are suspended in liquid – the medication is not dissolved. In order to help the medication stay equally suspended (distributed throughout the liquid), an agent is added to make the preparation thick. Nevertheless, given enough time, ingredients settle and collect at the bottom of bottles. You must shake stock bottles of suspensions before dispensing them. It is also necessary that you put "Shake Well" auxiliary labels on patients' prescription containers.

Reconstituting powders to liquids requires the addition of a specific amount of distilled water to convert them into solutions or suspensions. Because these medications deteriorate rapidly as liquids, they are manufactured and stored as dry powders. Distilled water is added to them immediately before they are dispensed. After reconstituting, these medications generally are effective for 10 to 14 days, and they usually need to be refrigerated. Many liquid antibiotics fall into this category.

Elixirs are clear, hydroalcoholic (combinations of water and alcohol) liquids intended for oral use. They often contain flavoring substances.

Fluid extracts and tinctures use alcohol, water, or combinations of the two as their base and usually contain plant extracts as active ingredients.

Spirits or essences are alcoholic or hydroalcoholic solutions of volatile substances. They contain such a high percentage of alcohol that they require storage in tight containers to prevent loss through evaporation.

Syrups are concentrated solutions of sugar in water with active ingredients. They may also contain alcohol.

Emulsions are mixtures of oil and water. Given enough time, they usually separate into an oil layer on top and a water layer on the bottom. Therefore, you must shake stock bottles of emulsions before dispensing them. It is also necessary that you put "Shake Well" auxiliary labels on patients' prescription containers.

Topical Dosage Forms

Certain liquids are used as topical treatments (i.e., outside the body, as opposed to "internal" or inside the body). Most of these are used to treat the eyes, ears, and skin. In addition, the vaginal and rectal areas are considered "topical areas;" hence, creams, and suppositories are delivered to these areas through the use of special applicators. Following is a description of the most common topical dosage forms:

Ointments are greasy preparations, usually with a petroleum jelly base. They are good for delivering medication to areas of the skin that need protection. Ointments leave oily coatings on skin.

Creams are combinations of water, oil, and other substances. They usually do not offer as much protection as ointments, but they are more appealing to patients because creams are less greasy and are usually absorbed by the skin.

Lotions are like creams, but they contain more liquid and are applied more easily over larger areas of the body.

Liniments are mixtures of various substances in oil, alcoholic solutions of soap, or emulsions intended for external application. They are often used for their heat-producing effects.

Gels are semisolid suspensions of very small particles, usually in a water base.

Collodions are liquids that dry as flexible films on skin. Many wart, corn, or callous removers are prepared as collodions.

Transdermal patches are recently-developed topical delivery systems designed for prolonged action. Medications are provided in patches that, like Band-Aid strips, stick to skin with adhesives. When patches are applied, the skin absorbs constant amounts of medication over a time period ranging from 12 hours to several days. Examples of medications used in transdermal patches are nitroglycerin for angina, estrogens for hormone replacement, and nicotine to help people stop smoking.

Suppositories are topical dosage forms. Usually manufactured in cylindrical, egg, or pear shapes, some are made for insertion into the rectum; others into the vagina. Medication is absorbed into the body through this route or has local effects.

Vaginal tablets are inserted into the vagina. Whenever typing directions for using vaginal tablets or suppositories, remind patients to remove any outer wrapping, such as aluminum foil, before inserting.

Otic and ophthalmic preparations are also considered topical dosage forms. Otic (ear) medications are usually supplied in dropper bottles; ophthalmic (eye) preparations may be drops or ointments. Ophthalmic medications must be sterile (i.e., free of bacterial contamination).

Miscellaneous Dosage Forms

Aerosols are sprayable products that use pressurized gas and valve systems to deliver medications. They are most commonly used for topical application to skin or for inhalation into the lungs and nasal passages.

Chewing gum is also used to administer medication. With this method, medications are absorbed through the mouth's mucous membranes. The most common example of this dosage form, Nicorette gum, delivers nicotine to help people stop smoking.

Parenteral medications are sterile preparations injected with syringes. Insulin is the most common parenteral medicine stocked in community pharmacies.

PRESCRIPTION CONTAINERS

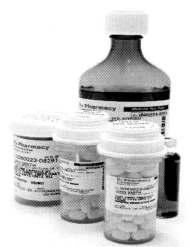

Containers used to dispense medications come in various types, shapes, and sizes. The various types of containers are described below, followed by a description of the special child-resistant containers (i.e., caps) used for vials and bottles.

Examples of prescription containers.

Containers

Vials. These cylinder-shaped plastic containers are used when dispensing tablets or capsules. Because light causes medication to deteriorate faster, vials are amber in color to protect the contents from the destructive effects of sunlight and artificial light.

Ointment jars. These plastic or glass jars hold ointments and creams. Like vials, ointment jars are opaque to protect their contents from light.

Bottles. Liquid medications are dispensed in glass or plastic, amber-colored prescription bottles to protect them from light. The bottle's size is generally indicated by a Roman numeral near the top of its back (flat) side. Therefore, if you need a container that holds 4 fluid ounces you would look for a container with the letters "iv" embossed on it. Bottles for liquid medications generally come in the following sizes:

- 2 fluid ounces: ii
- 4 fluid ounces: iv
- 6 fluid ounces: vi
- 8 fluid ounces: viii
- 12 fluid ounces: xii
- 16 fluid ounces: xvi

Like household measuring cups, prescription bottles have marks on either side of them to indicate fluid ounces and milliliters. Ounces are embossed in one-half ounce increments on the left-hand side of the back of the bottle. Milliliters are marked in increments of 10 ml on the right-hand side of the back of the bottle. Prescription bottles have a raised line on the neck's back that indicates when they are full. Do not over-fill the bottle; the patient may spill the contents when taking the cap off. Bottle markings are approximates but are usually sufficient to measure a single ingredient for dispensing.

Dropper bottles. These amber glass bottles have droppers attached to the inside of their caps. Dropper bottles are available in various sizes and hold liquid medications that are taken a few drops at a time.

Applicator bottles. Made of amber glass, these containers have slender, clear-glass or plastic rods attached to the inside of their caps. The rods have bulb-like ends which act as applicators for liquids. Patients dip the rod into the medication and dab the bulb onto the affected area of their skin.

Closures

Closures (caps) for vials and bottles come in two styles: child-resistant or easy-open. Some child-resistant caps must be simultaneously pushed down and twisted – a task requiring more coordination than most young children have. All prescription medications are dispensed in vials with child-resistant caps unless patients or prescribers request otherwise. Some elderly or disabled patients find child-resistant caps difficult to open. If there are no young children in the home, patients may choose not to receive child-resistant containers in favor of simple easy-open caps. With such requests, you should ask patients to sign a document, which is kept on file, authorizing the use of easy-open caps.

Some medications are never dispensed in child-resistant packages because patients must be able to administer them immediately, especially in life-threatening situations. Other products are dispensed to patients in original packages and do not require child-resistant closures: those requiring a special glass container, those allowing only a certain quantity per package, or those packaged specially, such as oral contraceptives.

The following list includes the generic and brand names of the most common medications that do not need to be dispensed in child-resistant containers.

- isosorbide dinitrate sublingual and chewable forms (e.g., Isordil®)
- oral contraceptives in unit-of-use packages
- cholestyramine powder (e.g., Questran®)
- potassium powders and tablets in packets (e.g., K-Lyte®)
- methylprednisolone tablets in unit-of-use packages (e.g., Medrol Dosepak®)
- mebendazole unit dose tablets (e.g., Vermox®)
- metered-dose inhalers such as: Proventil®, Ventolin® (albuterol sulfate); Alupent® (metaproterenol sulfate); Vancenase®, Beconase® (beclomethasone dipropionate)

It is important to remember that nitroglycerin sublingual tablets must be dispensed in the original, unopened container, labeled with the following statement directed to the patient: "Warning: to prevent loss of potency, keep these tablets in the original container or in a supplemental Nitroglycerin container specifically labeled as being suitable for Nitroglycerin Tablets. Close tightly immediately after each use."

> **Note:** Many pharmacies have adopted policies and procedures for handling requests for prescriptions without safety closures. For more information about special packaging, ask your pharmacist supervisor.

GENERIC PRODUCTS

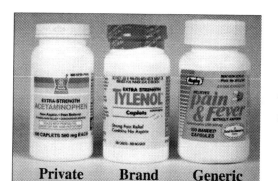

Three examples of acetaminophen extra-strength products

Private Label   Brand Name   Generic Company

Every medication has a "Generic name," the official or chemical name of the product's active ingredients. "Aspirin" is an example of a generic drug product name. **Some** medications **also** have "brand names," the trademarked name given to products by manufacturers. The term "trade name" is also used for these products. "Bayer®" or "Anacin®" are examples of two brand names or trade names used for aspirin products.

Drug products that are available from more than one manufacturer are called "multiple-source" drugs. Multiple-source drugs that do not have brand names are commonly called "Generic drugs," "generic equivalents," or "generics."

Some drug products are not available as generics. The main reason for this is that most new products are developed under a patent. Patents expire in approximately 17 years from the time of discovery of the drug—not from the time the product is available for sale. This exclusivity gives companies incentives to invest in research and develop new products. With patent protection periods, manufacturers are more likely to recover their investments. Once patents expire, competing companies may sell generic versions of a medication.

Generics are usually sold for less than their brand-name equivalents. This lower price has led some people to think that generics are in some way inferior to brand-name products. Actually, the Food and Drug Administration (FDA) requires that generics meet the same quality standards as brand-name products. Generic drug manufacturers need to demonstrate **pharmaceutical equivalence** (same active ingredients, same dosage form, same route of administration, and same strength) as well as **therapeutic equivalence** (same rate and extent of absorption of the active ingredients into the bloodstream) to the brand name drug.

Before deciding whether to select a brand-name or generic product, pharmacists consider patients' needs, the potential savings from the generic, and whether there is a wide range between the medication's effective dosage and its toxic dosage. Occasionally, pharmacists may prefer brand-name products over generics when they feel it is in patients' best interests. Examples of some multiple-source products that some pharmacists do not substitute include: Coumadin® (warfarin sodium); Dilantin® (phenytoin sodium); Lanoxin® (digoxin); and Synthroid® (levothyroxine sodium).

Although there are some exceptions, pharmacists usually prefer to dispense generics because:
- Generics save patients money, sometimes allowing them to obtain prescriptions they could not afford otherwise.
- Generics help the pharmacy keep prescription prices competitive.
- Generics are sometimes required by third-party insurance programs. Patients who wish to receive brand-name products for multiple-source medications may be required by third-party payers to pay a larger portion of the prescription cost.

Dispensing Multiple-Source Products

Each state regulates the circumstances under which generic medications may be substituted. Some states prohibit generic substitution unless specifically authorized by prescribers; others permit pharmacists to substitute generic equivalents unless prescribers specifically prohibit it. Examples of various states' requirements are listed below:

- Some states have two boxes on prescription forms that prescribers may check to either permit or forbid substitution.

- Some states require two signature lines on prescription forms: one line for "generics permitted" and one for "brand name only." Prescribers sign on one of these lines to indicate dispensing instructions.

- Prescribers can only prevent substitution in some states by writing on the prescription form in their own handwriting, "Dispense As Written" (DAW), "Brand Medically Necessary," or "No Substitution" (NS).

- Many states require pharmacists to offer patients generic products when available. In some states, posted signs explaining the availability of generics are considered sufficient notice.

Your state may enforce certain labeling requirements for multiple-source products. Generally, when dispensing a generic product, the generic name of the medication must appear on the prescription label. Check with a pharmacist about your state's regulations.

Many pharmacy departments stock only one generic equivalent for each brand-name medication even though several equivalent generics may be available. You should learn your state's requirements and your pharmacy's policies and procedures regarding product selection and work under the pharmacist's supervision to help assure compliance with these requirements.

The Orange Book

The Orange Book, officially titled *Approved Drug Products with Therapeutic Equivalence Evaluations*, lists bioequivalence ratings for prescription and over-the-counter drug products that have received FDA approval for safety and effectiveness. It is the basis for generic product evaluation and selection by pharmacists and prescribers. *The Orange Book* defines the following terms:

Pharmaceutical equivalents - medications that have the same active ingredients, the same dosage form, same route of administration and same strength. They may differ with regard to shape, color, packaging and inactive ingredients.

Pharmaceutical alternatives are medications that have the same therapeutic moiety but may differ with regard to the particular chemical complex, salt or ester of the product or may differ with regard to dosage form or strength. Examples of products that are pharmaceutical alternatives but not pharmaceutical equivalents are Tylenol® tablets vs. Tylenol® capsules; ferrous sulfate vs. ferrous gluconate and amoxicillin 250 mg capsules vs. amoxicillin 500 mg capsules.

Therapeutic equivalents are medications that are pharmaceutical equivalents AND have the same clinical effect and safety profile. These products are also said to be generic equivalents and can be substituted for each other subject to the requirements of the various states. In the *Orange Book*, these products are designated by the letter "A" or A-rated. If a product is not generically equivalent, they are designated by the letter "B" or B-rated. For example, Plavix® 75 mg tablets and clopidogrel 75 mg tablets are therapeutically equivalent and therefore are A-rated.

Therapeutic alternatives are medications that do not have the same active ingredients but have similar clinical effects. These products are also said to be therapeutic alternatives. Zantac® (ranitidine) and Pepcid® (famotidine) are from the same therapeutic drug class (H-2 antagonists for treatment of ulcers) and are considered therapeutic alternatives. Some hospital formulary systems allow substitution of therapeutic alternatives. Community pharmacies, however, are not allowed to make therapeutic substitutions without specific authorization of the prescriber.

Most Frequently Prescribed Medications

The Appendix contains a list of the 200 most frequently prescribed medications. Included in the listing are brand-name medications as well as generic drugs. The drug products included in this list represent the medications you should try to learn as soon as possible.

STOCK BOTTLE LABELS

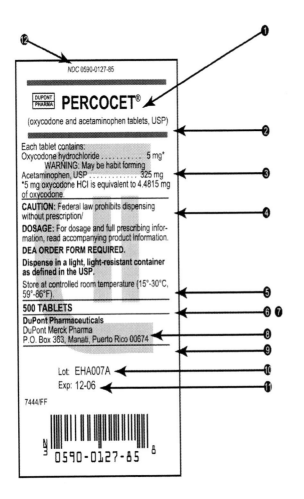

Medications arrive from your supplier in the manufacturer's packaging, called "stock bottles." The FDA requires all prescription medication stock bottle labels to contain the following information:

❶ The brand name or trade name. The manufacturer may use a trade name, especially for multiple-source products. As explained previously, not all products are given brand names.

❷ The generic name. All medications have a generic name, the official or chemical name of the product's active ingredients. Brand-name medications can also be referred to by their generic names. For example the OTC decongestant, Sudafed® also has its generic name, "pseudoephedrine".

❸ The medication's strength. This indicates the amount of the active ingredient. Many medications are available in different strengths, which must be clearly visible on the label. If a product is a combination of two or more products, each ingredient and its strength must be listed on the label.

❹ The legend statement. Medications that can be dispensed only by prescription must have either an "Rx only" symbol or the following statement (or legend) on their labels: "Caution: Federal law prohibits dispensing without a prescription." For this reason, prescription-only medications are also known as "legend drugs." Never stock medications with this legend or the "Rx only" symbol in areas accessible to patients.

5   **Storage requirements.** Most, but not all, medications can be stored at room temperature. Medications should not be subjected to or stored in extreme hot or cold conditions because this can cause them to break down or lose potency. Some medications require refrigeration, either from the time of manufacture, or from the time they are dispensed to the patient. Insulin is refrigerated from the time it is manufactured. Other medications, such as antibiotic suspensions, need to be refrigerated only after water is added to the powder in the manufacturer's bottle at the time the medication is dispensed to the patient. Manufacturers' labels indicate how products should be stored.

6   **The package quantity.** Many prescription medications are available in many pack-age sizes. The quantities of products other than tablets and capsules, are expressed in both the household and metric units. For example, 16 fl. ounces or 473 mL.

7   **The medication's dosage form.** The dosage form is identified as tablet, capsule, topical ointment, liquid suspension, etc. The label will indicate the intended method of administration. For example, topical products say "for external use only." Eye products say "for ophthalmic use only."

8   **The manufacturer's name.** The manufacturer's name must be on the label. In the case of generics, the distributor's name may also be given.

9   **The controlled substance mark.** If medications are classified as controlled substances, (i.e., Schedule II-V medications) manufacturers' labels must indicate this with a "C" and the Roman numeral classification assigned by the DEA to describe its level of control (e.g., C-II). This symbol will appear in the upper right corner of the label or the symbol may be overprinted in a contrasting color.

10   **The lot number.** Sometimes called a "control number," this number marks medications as belonging to particular batches produced by the manufacturer. In the event that products manufactured at a particular time are recalled, they are identified by lot number.

11   **The expiration date.** When manufactured, every prescription medication is given an expiration date. If only the month and year are listed, the expiration date is the last date of the month. The time period between the date of manufacture and the expiration date is called the shelf-life. The shelf-life is the period during which properly stored, unopened packages of medication can be sold because their potency is still expected to be intact. Potency is not assured after the expiration date. Expired medications should be removed from stock and, if possible, returned according to your pharmacy's policies and procedures.

The NDC number. The National Drug Code (NDC) number is assigned by the manufacturer and placed on all prescription stock packages. Each package size has its own NDC number which gives three pieces of information about the medication:

1. The first five digits identify the manufacturer

2. The next four digits identify the name, strength and dosage form of the medication

3. The last two digits identify the package size

For example, for the NDC number: 00004 – 0169 – 49

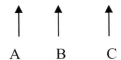

A is the manufacturer: Roche Laboratories, in this case
B is the product: Accutane®, 20 mg capsules
C is the size of this package: 100 capsules/package

NDC numbers are often used by pharmacy computer systems to designate the medication dispensed and to complete third-party billing.

> **Note:** Whenever you write NDC numbers (for example, on third-party claim forms), all leading zeroes must be added. The numbers must have 11 digits in the pattern shown above: five digits, then four digits, then two digits. The zeros act as place-holders. For example, if the NDC number contains only four digits in the manufacturer section, a zero is added to the beginning. If there are only three digits in the product section, a zero is added to the beginning. If the dosage section has only one digit, a zero is again added at the beginning.
>
> Add any necessary leading zeroes so that the NDC number contains 11 digits.

DISTINGUISHING AMONG EASILY-CONFUSED PRODUCTS

Watch out for medication names that look or sound alike. It is easy to confuse the names of these medications when they are written or spoken. When you receive prescriptions from patients, always check with a pharmacist to make sure you have identified the correct product. At the end of this chapter, you will find a list of medications with names that look or sound alike. Familiarize yourself with this list.

No matter how careful and accurate you are, there are products that lend themselves to dispensing errors. Here is a short list of some of these products:

- **Hydroxyzine and Hydralazine.** Both drug names sound alike with the first four letters and the last four letters of each name being identical. The proximity of both these drugs on the pharmacy shelves also contribute to dispensing the incorrect product. Differentiate the drug names by using boldface, color, and/or "tall man" letters (e.g., hydrOXYzine, hydrALAzine).

- **Humalog® and Humulin®, Novolin® 70/30 and Novolog® Mix 70/30.** Similar names, strengths, and concentration add to the confusion and contribute to medication errors. Familiarize yourself with the different types of insulin to identify potential errors.

- **Metformin and Metronidazole.** Potentially for serious mix-ups were linked with look-alike packaging or selection of the wrong drug in the computer when entering the mnemonic "met500." Use vigilance in selecting and dispensing the drug.

- **Hydromorphone injection and morphine injection.** These products are sometimes though to be generic equivalents, however they are not interchangeable. Substitution can lead to overdose or increased side effects. Both injections come in similar concentrations.

- **OxyContin® and oxycodone.** The assumption is made that these two medications are the same because they are both oxycodone. However, OxyContin® is a extended release formulation while oxycodone is an immediately release tablet. Never make assumptions about brand and generic formulations.

Examples of Look-Alike or Sound-Alike Medication Names

Following are some medication names that may cause problems. Many were taken from lists published in *Pharmacy Times*, JCAHO, and FDA

Acetohexamide	acetazolamide
Advicor®	Advair®
Amicar®	Omacor®
Avinza®	Evista®
Bupropion	buspirone
Cardura®	Coumadin®
Celebrex®	Cerebyx®
Chlorpromazine	chlorpropamide
Clomiphene	clomipramine
Clonidine	Klonopin®
Cyclosporine	cycloserine
Daunorubicin	doxorubicin
Darvocet®	Percocet®
Diabeta®	Zebeta®
Diflucan®	Diprivan®
Dimenhydrinate	diphenhydramine
Dobutamine	dopamine
Effexor XR®	Effexor®
Ephedrine	epinephrine
folic acid	folinic Acid
Glipizide	glyburide
Heparin	Hespan®
Hydrocodone	oxycodone
Lamivudine	lamotrigine
Leukeran	leucovorin calcium
Methylprednisolone	methyltestosterone
MS Contin®	Oxycontin®
Mucinex®	Mucomyst®
Nicardipine	nifedipine
opium tincture	paregoric (camphorated opium tincture)
Prednisone	prednisolone
Prilosec	Prozac®
Retrovir®	Ritonavir®
Tizanidine	tiagabine
tolazamide	tolbutamide
Topamax®	Toprol XL®
Tramadol®	trazadone
vinblastine	vincristine
Wellbutrin SR®	Wellbutrin XL®
Zantac®	Xanax®
Zantac®	Zyrtec®
Zestril®	Zyprexa®
Zestril®	Zetia®
Zocor®	Zyrtec®

PUBLIC SAFETY

Although the FDA is very thorough in the approval process of a medication, it is impossible to fully prove that a drug is safe for use. Pharmacy technicians can play a very important role in promoting safe medication use by being familiar with several programs aimed at promoting public safety.

MedWatch

The FDA has initiated MedWatch as a voluntary reporting system for adverse effects or medication errors with pharmaceutical products. Serious problems suspected to be associated with drugs and medical devices can be reported online, by phone or by mailing or faxing a MedWatch form to the FDA. Safety alerts, recalls, withdrawals, and important labeling changes are distributed to the medical community and the general public via the FDA Enforcement Report or online at www.fda.gov.

The FDA has several options if it determines that a marketed drug presents a risk of illness, injury or gross consumer deception. It may then decide to seek an injunction that would prevent the manufacturer from distributing the drug, seize the drug, or issue a recall. If you are aware of an adverse effect of a drug or potential medication errors that could be prevented by better packaging, labeling, etc. please encourage the pharmacist to fill out a MedWatch report.

Drug Recalls

When the FDA receives enough reports of adverse effects or misbranding that it decides the product is a threat to the public health, it contacts the manufacturer and recommends a recall.

The FDA classifies drug recalls three ways depending on the type of adverse effects:

Class I: A drug product is being recalled because there is a strong chance of serious adverse effects or death to the patient.

Class II: A drug product is being recalled because there is a temporary (but reversible) chance of adverse effect, or little chance of serious adverse effect.

Class III: A drug product is being recalled because of some problem that is not likely to cause adverse effects.

If the manufacturer agrees to a recall, it must establish a recall strategy with the FDA that addresses the depth of the recall, the extent of public warnings, and a means for checking the effectiveness of the recall. The depth of the recall is identified by wholesaler, retailer, or consumer levels. The effectiveness may require anything from no follow-up, to complete checks via phone calls, letters, or in person.

When there is a drug recall, the pharmacist may ask you to remove selected products from the inventory and prepare them to be returned to a manufacturer or wholesaler. Patients may hear about the recall from news reports and may have questions. Be sure to refer these questions to the pharmacist but do not say anything to patients that may alarm them.

Pregnancy Category

The FDA requires that each drug product be classified in one of five pregnancy categories intended to help prescribers and patients with decisions about drug therapy for pregnant women or those who may become pregnant. The categories reflect the potential of a systemically absorbed drug to cause birth defects:

<u>Category A</u>:   Studies in pregnant women failed to show a risk to the fetus; fetal harm appears remote

<u>Category B</u>:   Either animal studies have shown no risk, but controlled studies in pregnant women are not done, or animal studies have shown an adverse effect that was not confirmed in women

<u>Category C</u>:   Either animal studies have shown an effect on the fetus & there are no controlled trials in women, or there are not studies in either animals or women; should be given only if the benefits to the fetus outweigh the risks

<u>Category D</u>:   There is positive evidence of risk to a human fetus; must weigh the risks versus the benefits

<u>Category X</u>:   There are studies to show fetal abnormalities; the drug is contraindicated in women who may be pregnant

If your pharmacy computer system alerts you about a Category D or Category X product for a woman of childbearing age, be sure that the pharmacist is aware of this potential problem. You might also want to ask your pharmacist for a list of drug products most commonly associated with birth defects.

SELF-ASSESSMENT QUESTIONS CHAPTER II

1. Sublingual tablets are:
   a. Intended to be chewed before swallowing.
   b. Placed under the tongue.
   c. Placed in the area between the cheek and gums.
   d. Coated to prevent them from dissolving in the stomach.

2. Which of the following liquid dosage forms contain a mixture of oil and water?
   a. Spirits.
   b. Elixirs.
   c. Emulsions.
   d. Suspensions.

3. Which of the following statements is TRUE of child-resistant closures?
   a. Child-resistant closures are required by the Food and Drug Administration.
   b. Only patients may request not to receive child-resistant closures.
   c. Nitroglycerin sublingual tablets are not required to be dispensed in bottles with child-resistant closures.
   d. All prescription medications must be dispensed in child-resistant closures.

4. Which of the following is a piece of information indicated by the NDC number?
   a. The expiration date.
   b. The package size.
   c. The lot number
   d. The average wholesale price (AWP).

5. The name of the FDA program which encourages health care professionals to report adverse drug effects is:
   a. Medscape.
   b. MedWatch.
   c. MedLine.
   d. MedManage.

Answers: 1) b   2) c   3) c   4) b   5) b.

PHARMACY TECHNICIAN COMPETENCY ASSESSMENT CHAPTER II

Description of Ability or Skill	Initials		Training Completed	
	Tech	R.Ph.	Date	Remarks
The technician trainee is familiar with the characteristics of and can cite examples from each of the four major categories of dosage forms.				
The technician trainee is familiar with the characteristics of and can cite examples of prescription containers and closures.				
The technician trainee can identify and locate in the pharmacy department several different sizes and styles of prescription containers and the closures appropriate for each.				
The technician trainee understands and can explain what generic drugs are and how they compare to brand-name medications.				
The technician trainee can describe the state's rules regarding the substitution of generic equivalents as well as the pharmacy department's policies concerning such substitutions.				

PHARMACY TECHNICIAN COMPETENCY ASSESSMENT CHAPTER II

| Description of Ability or Skill | Initials | | Training Completed | |
	Tech	R.Ph.	Date	Remarks
The technician trainee can identify the types of information found on medication stock bottles.				
The technician trainee can describe strategies for avoiding mix-ups among easily-confused products.				

Chapter III
Prescription Medications –
Controlled Substances

EDUCATIONAL OBJECTIVES

After studying the material in this chapter, the technician trainee should be able to:

- Differentiate among the various controlled substances schedules and rules for filing controlled-substance prescriptions
- Understand the rules and regulations governing refills, partial refills, and transfers of controlled substances
- Follow the correct procedures for handling Schedule V sales

CONTROLLED SUBSTANCES

The Drug Enforcement Administration (DEA) regulates controlled substances—drugs that have potential for abuse or physical or psychological dependence. Each state also regulates controlled substances through state boards of pharmacy or, sometimes, through another state agency.

Note: If regulations governing scheduled medications in your state differ from the federal regulations, the stricter regulations must be followed.

Classification of Controlled Substances

Controlled substances are classified by federal law into five schedules. These schedules are referred to in either of two ways:

- Schedule I   or   C-I
- Schedule II   or   C-II
- Schedule III   or   C-III
- Schedule IV   or   C-IV
- Schedule V   or   C-V

	Refills	Partial Fills	Storage	Rx needed	Ordering	Filing	Stocked in Pharmacy
			Comparison of Prescriptions for Scheduled and Non-Scheduled Medications[2]				
C-I	-	-	-	-	-	-	No
C-II	None	Remainder in 72 hr	Locked safe	Yes Must be written	DEA Form 222	Filed separately	Yes
C-III	As directed up to 5 times within 6 months	Remainder before Rx expires	Locked safe or dispersed with regular stock	Yes	Regular order form	Filed with C-IV & V only or marked with red "C" and filed with non-controlled Rxs	Yes
C-IV	As directed up to 5 times within 6 months	Remainder before Rx expires	Locked safe or dispersed with regular stock	Yes	Regular order form	Filed with C-III & V only or marked with red "C" and filed with non-controlled Rxs	Yes
C-V	Depends[3]	If Rx required, remainder before Rx expires	Regular stock	Some require Rx; some are OTC. Also varies by state[4]	Regular order form	If Rx required: filed with C-III & IV only or marked with red "C" and filed with non-controlled Rxs	Yes
Non-controlled Rx	As directed up to one year.	Remainder before Rx expires	Regular stock	Yes	Regular order form	Filed separately or marked with red "C" and filed with C-III-V Rxs	Yes

[2] Federal law may be different than state law for controlled substance. This table focuses only on federal law. Ask your pharmacist for more information about state laws concerning controlled substances.
[3] Products are subject to sales restriction depending on the product and max allowable limit determined by state. Ask your pharmacist for more information.
[4] Some states require prescriptions for Schedule V Controlled Substances. Ask the pharmacist for more information.

The five federal schedules are as follows:

Schedule I (C-I) includes drugs that have a high potential for abuse, no currently accepted medical use in the United States, and are unsafe for use under medical supervision. These products are not found in pharmacy departments. Examples are LSD and heroin.

Schedule II (C-II) includes medications having a currently accepted medical use in the United States and a high potential for abuse and physical or psychological dependence. Some examples are morphine (a narcotic), methamphetamine (a stimulant), and secobarbital (a sedative).

Schedule III (C-III) includes medications that have an abuse potential less than that of medications listed in Schedules I and II. Abuse of these medications may lead to moderate or low physical dependence or high psychological dependence. One example is Tylenol⁻ with Codeine No.3. Certain stimulants or depressants are also included in Schedule III.

Schedule IV (C-IV) medications have less potential for abuse than Schedule I, II, or III medications. Abuse of these medications may lead to only a limited physical or psychological dependence. Examples include phenobarbital, Valium, and Xanax.

Schedule V (C-V) medications have low potential for abuse and limited physical or psychological dependence. Schedule V medications are any compound, mixture or preparation containing a limited amount of a controlled substance in combination with non-controlled active ingredients. These products are generally used as cough suppressants or as antidiarrheals. Some examples include Novahistine Expectorant and Lomotil.

Dispensing Controlled-Substance Prescriptions

Schedule I substances are never stocked in pharmacies. In fact, it is illegal in the United States to possess these substances.

Schedule II medications are only dispensed on written prescriptions personally signed by the prescribers. Schedule II prescriptions **must** be typed or handwritten in ink. They **must** contain the full name and address of the patient, the date of issue, and the medication information. Federal law allows a facsimile to serve as the original written prescription for long-term care facility (LTCF) residents or for hospice patients. Schedule II narcotic prescriptions for parenteral use by a home infusion pharmacy can also be faxed. Since some states may not allow prescriptions for Schedule II medications to be faxed, you should ask your pharmacist supervisor whether this is allowed in your state.

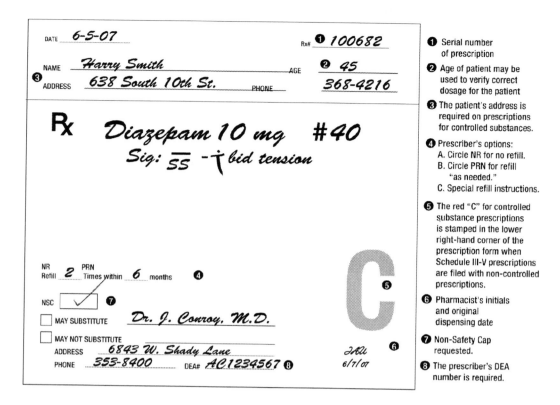

An example of a prescription for a Schedule IV controlled substance.

Some states have additional regulations such as writing the quantity in words as well as numbers, making duplicate or triplicate copies of the prescription, and limiting the time during which the prescription may be dispensed. In the case of duplicate and triplicate forms, a copy of each Schedule II prescription must be sent to the appropriate state or government agency, usually each month. When the prescription has been dispensed, a pharmacist usually cancels the prescription form by drawing a line across its face, dating, and signing or initialing the prescription form.

Depending on your state's policy, you may need to confirm patients' identities when dispensing Schedule II medications. Ask to see a driver's license or ask patients to sign the prescription form. Some pharmacy department policies require pharmacists to call prescribers to confirm orders for Schedule II medications.

Sometimes, only a limited amount of a C-II medication may be dispensed to patients. Some states allow the dispensing of a one-month supply. Check with a pharmacist about your state's rules and regulations.

- **Partial filling of C-II medications.** Because pharmacy departments stock small amounts of Schedule II medications, you may only be able to partially fill these prescriptions. When this happens, a pharmacist must note the partial quantity dispensed on the face of the prescription order. A new supply of the medication must be ordered, and the remainder of the prescription must be filled **within 72 hours** of the partial filling. Pharmacists may also transfer the needed quantity from another pharmacy, providing the proper recordkeeping is completed. If your pharmacy fails to fill the balance of the prescription within the time limit (72 hours), a pharmacist must call the prescriber to request a new prescription. Federal regulations allow exceptions to the restrictions on a partial filling of C-II medications for patients in a long term care facility or for patients with a terminal illness. Check with your pharmacist supervisor about the requirements on partial filling of C-II medications.

- **Emergency prescriptions for C-II medications.** In emergencies, prescriptions for C-II medication may be phoned in by prescribers. Verbal prescriptions for C-II medications may only be received by a pharmacist, and it is a pharmacist's responsibility to assure that phoned-in prescriptions are legitimate.

  Only the amount needed to treat the patient during the emergency may be dispensed. Prescribers are required to furnish the pharmacy with a written, signed prescription order for the emergency dispensing within seven days. Some states, however, are stricter and require that a written prescription be obtained within 72 hours. Check with your pharmacist supervisor about the requirements in your state.

- **Refilling C-II medications.** Schedule II medications may not be refilled under any circumstances. If a patient needs more medication, the prescriber must write a new prescription.

- **Storing C-II medications.** Federal regulations require Schedule II medications to be stored so they are difficult to steal. There are a variety of ways to do this, and acceptable methods of storage differ from state to state. The most secure method is to keep Schedule II medications in a locked safe. A locked cabinet is also acceptable in some states.

  Many states allow pharmacy departments to disperse C-II medications in with their regular stock. Check with a pharmacist about your pharmacy department's method of complying with the law.

- **Ordering Schedule II medications.** All Schedule II medication orders and invoices must be separately maintained. Any order for a Schedule II medication must be placed on government-issued Schedule II DEA Order Forms (i.e., DEA Form 222).

  All transfers of Schedule II medications between pharmacy departments must be recorded on this form. These medication records are kept separately so they can be easily tracked.

Only pharmacists are authorized to complete and sign the form. Typically, the pharmacist will fill out, sign, and date the form on the day the pharmacy department places the order. When the Schedule II order arrives, a pharmacist will check that the quantity and amounts ordered match those received and log them in on the order form.

- **Perpetual inventory of C-II medications.** Some states require a perpetual (constant) inventory of Schedule II medications. Many pharmacy departments choose to keep a perpetual inventory, even when not required by law. This "running" inventory record immediately informs pharmacists if controlled substances are missing or unaccounted for. The perpetual inventory shows when new bottles containing Schedule II medications are added to stock, when and how much medication is removed from stock bottles to fill prescriptions, and the amount of product remaining in stock bottles. Very often the pharmacy computer is used to automatically calculate these transactions.

> **Note:** In addition, the DEA rules and regulations require a separate, manual inventory be conducted every two years to track all controlled substances. Inventories can be taken more often than required by law.

Schedules III and IV. Written, faxed (if allowed by your state), and oral prescription orders are permissible and prescriptions for these substances may be refilled up to five times within six months after the prescription's date of issue, if authorized by the prescriber.

Schedule V. Whenever a prescription is **not** required for the sale of a Schedule V medication, the purchaser and the dispenser must sign the "Schedule V Records Log." However, some states will not allow the sale of Schedule V medications without a prescription. If you work in one of these states, patients will have to present a prescription to obtain the medication.

- **Pseudoephedrine Policy:** Effective January 15, 2006, the Methamphetamine Precursor Control Act (MPCA) makes pseudoephedrine and ephedrine "Schedule V controlled substances." The law places ephedrine, pseudoephedrine, and phenylpropanolamine into a new Controlled Substances Act category. Drugs containing these products are subject to sales restrictions, storage requirements, and record-keeping requirements. If your state has requirements that are more strict than the federal act, the stronger requirements take precedence. Be sure to ask your pharmacist supervisor about the requirements in your state. The new federal law only applies to over-the-counter products and not prescription medications. The law creates a sales limit of 3.6 grams per day and 9 grams per month. (Mobile sellers have a limit of 7.5 grams per month.) The law also requires pharmacies to maintain a sales logbook. This logbook must contain the following information: product name, quantity sold, names and addresses of purchasers, and dates and times of the sales. The purchaser must present a photo ID prior to all sales. Maintaining a logbook may not be necessary in some instances. For example, gas stations are not required to maintain a logbook when selling single pseudoephedrine tablets.

The following information must be provided in a bound *Schedule V Records Log* (see below):

- Dispensing date
- Name of the product dispensed
- Quantity dispensed
- Name, signature and address of the purchaser
- Pharmacist's signature

Schedule-V Sales Record						
Date	Signature of Purchaser	Address of Purchaser	Name of Purchaser	Name of Product Sold	Quantity of Product Sold	Pharmacist's Signature

A sample page from a Schedule V Sales Record Log.

Following are some of the regulations regarding the dispensing of C-V medications:

- Only pharmacists can authorize sales of non-prescription Schedule V medications.
- However, pharmacy department clerks and technicians can complete the cash or
- credit transaction or deliver the product.
- The purchaser must be at least 18 years old.
- In most cases, Schedule V cough medicines are limited to four ounces per patient within a 48-hour period. Products containing opium for the control of diarrhea are limited to eight ounces per patient within a 48-hour period.
- When pharmacists are not familiar with patients, they must ask for identification.

Ask a pharmacist if your state has additional restrictions on the sale of Schedule V medications.

GENERAL REGULATIONS FOR CONTROLLED SUBSTANCES

Partial filling of C-III, C-IV, and C-V substances. If your pharmacy department does not have enough of a Schedule III, IV, or V medication in stock to completely fill a prescription, you may partially fill the order. The following guidelines must be followed:

- The partial dispensing must be recorded in the same manner as a refill.
- The total quantity dispensed in all partial fillings cannot exceed the total quantity prescribed.
- Medication may not be dispensed after the prescription expires (i.e., six months after the date of issue).

Transfer of C-III, C-IV, and C-V prescriptions to another pharmacy. In some cases, pharmacists may transfer a C-III, C-IV, and C-V prescription from one pharmacy department to another. After the prescription has been transferred to another pharmacy department, the pharmacist will make a note in the computer that the prescription has been transferred. This information should include the name of pharmacist, date transferred, DEA number, etc.

Ordinarily, scheduled prescriptions may be transferred only once; however, federal law allows pharmacies that share a real-time, on-line electronic database to transfer prescription refill information for Schedule III, IV and V substances as often as refills are authorized. Since the laws in some states may vary from federal law, consult with your pharmacist supervisor. Conversely, a prescription **received** as a transfer from another pharmacy department will have the word "Transfer" written across its face. The receiving pharmacy must obtain the last refill date and the dates and locations of all previous refills.

> **Note:** Some states require the pharmacy to receive new prescriptions from physicians and do not allow dispensing from a copy of a prescription transferred from another pharmacy.

Transfer of controlled substances between pharmacy departments. When pharmacies do not have a controlled substance in stock, some states allow pharmacists to obtain the medication from a second pharmacy department. Both pharmacy departments must keep a signed receipt of the transaction.

> **Note:** If the transfer involves a Schedule II medication, the official *DEA Order Form* (Form 222) must be completed and retained.

Prescription forms for C-II, C-III, C-IV, C-V substances. Prescription forms must contain the prescriber's address and DEA number, and the patient's address, along with all the standard information required for any prescription medication.

DEA NUMBER CHECK

Bogus DEA numbers on forged prescriptions may be detected by using the formula that the DEA created to generate DEA numbers. DEA numbers are composed of two letters followed by seven digits. The first letter is usually, but not always the letters A or B and the second letter must be the same as the first letter of the prescriber's last name.* DEA numbers commonly begin with M or F as well as A or B. There are four steps to checking the numerical portion of the DEA number. First, add the first, third, and fifth digits. Second, add the second, fourth and sixth digits and multiply the sum by two. Third, add the results of steps 1 and 2. Fourth, the last digit of the calculation should be the same as the seventh "check digit. Refer to the examples below.

Dr. Smith has the DEA number AS4967432
The first letter is A which checks because the first letter must be an A or B.
The second letter is S which checks because S is the first letter in Smith.
Next, the sum of the first, third, and fifth numbers is calculated.
$4 + 6 + 4 = 14$
Then, the product of the sum of the second, fourth, and sixth numbers is calculated.
$(9 + 7 + 3) \times 2$
$19 \times 2 = 38$
Finally, the sum of these two numbers is calculated and compared to the check digit.
$14 + 38 = 52$
The last number in 52 is 2 which is the last digit of the DEA number; therefore the DEA number follows DEA's formula.

Transfer warning statement. The following statement must be placed on the container for all prescribed controlled substances: **"Caution: Federal law prohibits transfer of this drug to any person other than the patient for whom it was prescribed."** This statement may be on an auxiliary label; sometimes it is pre-printed on the prescription label.

Filing prescription forms for controlled substances. Well-organized prescription files not only make verifying prescription information easy, they also will prepare you for audits. Your pharmacy department files could be inspected by a representative of the state board of pharmacy, or by the DEA.

---

*There are some exceptions. For example, a physician who changes her last name may retain an old DEA number.

Federal regulations for filing prescriptions require that:

- Schedule II prescription forms must be filed separately from all other prescription forms.

- Schedule III-V prescription forms must be "distinguishable" from all other prescription forms so they can be easily retrieved from general files. There are two options with regard to the filing and storage of the original prescription forms for Schedule III, IV, and V medications:

  1. The prescription forms may be filed with prescription forms for other non-controlled medications provided the forms for Schedule III, IV, and V medications are readily retrievable by a pharmacy's automatic data processing system or are stamped with a one-inch high red "C" in the lower right-hand corner. Some states, however, still require the red "C" to be stamped on the prescription. Ask your pharmacist supervisor to explain your state's requirements.

  2. The prescription forms for Schedule III, IV, and V medications may be filed in a third file separate from the file for C-II prescription forms and also separate from the file for prescription forms for non-controlled medication.

SELF-ASSESSMENT QUESTIONS CHAPTER III

1. Which schedule contains some medications that may be obtained without a prescription?
    a. C-II
    b. C-III
    c. C-IV
    d. C-V

2. According to <u>federal</u> law, inventories of controlled substances must be taken at least every
    a. month.
    b. six months.
    c. year.
    d. two years.

3. According to <u>federal</u> law, if an emergency prescription is received by telephone for a Schedule II drug, the prescriber must provide a written, signed prescription within:
    a. 2 days.
    b. 3 days.
    c. 4 days.
    d. 7 days.

4. In which controlled substance schedule is Tylenol with Codeine (acetaminophen/codeine) classified?
    a. C-II.
    b. C-III.
    c. C-IV.
    d. C-V.

Answers:
1) d
2) d
3) d
4) b

PHARMACY TECHNICIAN COMPETENCY ASSESSMENT
CHAPTER III

Description of Ability or Skill	Initials		Training Completed	
	Tech	R.Ph.	Date	Remarks
The technician trainee can differentiate among the various controlled-substances schedules.				
The technician trainee follows the proper rules and regulations when filing controlled-substance prescriptions.				
The technician trainee follows the proper rules and regulations when handling refills of controlled substances among pharmacies.				
The technician trainee follows the proper rules and regulations for partial filling of prescriptions for controlled substances.				
The technician trainee can describe the proper rules and regulations regarding transfers of prescriptions for controlled substances.				
The technician trainee can describe the correct procedures for handling Schedule V sales.				

Chapter IV
Prescriptions

EDUCATIONAL OBJECTIVES

After studying the material in this chapter, the technician trainee should be able to:

- List the professions which may prescribe medications
- List the information required on completed prescription forms
- Correctly translate prescribers' abbreviations and symbols into patient directions

---

Important Note

Although this chapter discusses laws and regulations related to prescribing authority by various practitioners and the requirements for receiving prescription facsimiles and transferring prescriptions, it should be noted that these laws and regulations vary from state to state. Ask your pharmacist supervisor for specific information about the requirements in your state.

PRESCRIBERS

Physicians (MD), dentists (DDS, DMD), osteopaths (DO), veterinarians (DVM), podiatrists (DPM) and, in some states, optometrists (OD) are authorized to prescribe prescription medications approved for use within these practitioners' areas of expertise. For example, dentists can prescribe medications pertaining to conditions affecting the mouth, gums, and teeth, including antibiotics, pain medications and a few other categories of prescription medications.

Some states permit physician assistants (PA), nurse practitioners (NP) and pharmacists (RPh or Pharm.D.) to prescribe certain medications according to specific guidelines. Additionally, some states allow medical interns, residents, and foreign doctors to prescribe medications under the authorization of a hospital or other health care institution in which they practice. These practitioners may be assigned a DEA number representing the institution's authorization for them to prescribe controlled substances.

Prescriber Signatures

Prescribers' signatures and addresses are required on all written prescriptions. Many signatures are difficult to read but, after a while, you will begin to recognize the signatures of prescribers whose patients frequently use the pharmacy where you work. Many prescription forms have prescribers' names and addresses preprinted on them. If you receive prescription forms with illegible names, ask patients for their prescribers' names and print them legibly on the prescription forms.

When you enter the prescriber's information into the computer, be sure you select the correct prescriber from the list the computer file offers you. Check that the prescriber's first name and address match those on the prescription. Printing wrong prescriber names on prescription labels can upset patients and can cause problems when they need prescriptions renewed.

RECEIVING PRESCRIPTIONS

Written Prescriptions

When you receive written prescriptions, quickly review them for completeness and legibility. The following information is typically found on prescriptions:

- The prescriber's name, address, and telephone number
- Patient's name
- Date prescription was issued
- Medication's name, strength, and dosage form or description of medical device
- Quantity to be dispensed
- Directions for use
- Number of refills permitted
- Whether generic substitution is permitted
- Prescriber's signature

The following information is required for all controlled substance prescriptions:

Patient's address
- Prescriber's DEA number

In addition, it is helpful if you can obtain the following information from the patient or the patient's representative if it is not already recorded in the patient profile:

- Patient's age or date of birth
- Patient's home and work telephone number

Remember that if medications come in only one strength or dosage form, that information need not be written on the prescription blank. If medications are available in two or more strengths and dosage forms, prescribers must specify what strength or dosage form patients should have. For example, the antibiotic amoxicillin is available as a suspension, a capsule and a chewable tablet. It also comes in three strengths: 125, 250 and 500 mg.

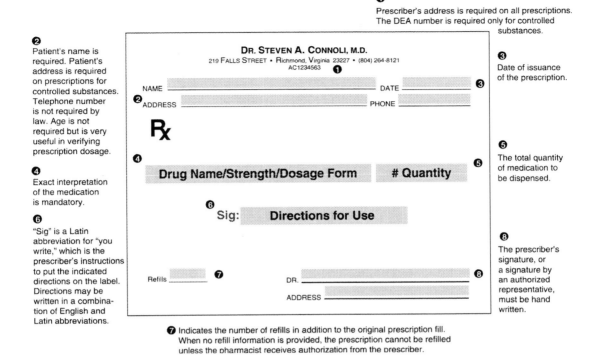

❶ Prescriber's address is required on all prescriptions. The DEA number is required only for controlled substances.

❷ Patient's name is required. Patient's address is required on prescriptions for controlled substances. Telephone number is not required by law. Age is not required but is very useful in verifying prescription dosage.

❸ Date of issuance of the prescription.

❹ Exact interpretation of the medication is mandatory.

❺ The total quantity of medication to be dispensed.

❻ "Sig" is a Latin abbreviation for "you write," which is the prescriber's instructions to put the indicated directions on the label. Directions may be written in a combination of English and Latin abbreviations.

❽ The prescriber's signature, or a signature by an authorized representative, must be hand written.

❼ Indicates the number of refills in addition to the original prescription fill. When no refill information is provided, the prescription cannot be refilled unless the pharmacist receives authorization from the prescriber.

The nine basic fields of information required for a complete prescription order.

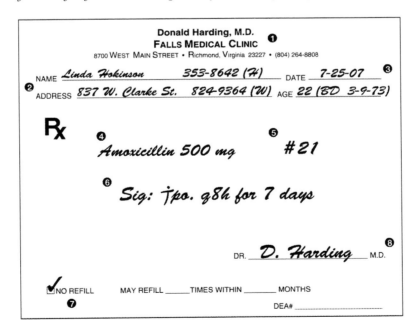

An example of a completed prescription form.

If this information is not provided on the prescription form, a pharmacist must call the prescriber to obtain it.

If refill information is not provided, you must assume no refills are authorized unless the pharmacist contacts the prescriber and receives permission to refill the prescription for a specified number of times.

The quantity to be dispensed can be described in several ways:
- Most commonly, quantity follows the # symbol.
- Occasionally, quantity is preceded by a prefix such as "Disp," an abbreviation for "Dispense."
- Sometimes quantity is preceded by the letters "DTD," a Latin abbreviation meaning "Give of such doses."
- The quantity itself may be written in words, (e.g., "two") Arabic numbers, (e.g., "2") or Roman numerals (e.g.,"ii").
- In some cases, the quantity may be incorporated with the patient directions, and you will have to calculate how much medication to dispense. For example, "One tablet three times daily for ten days," means that 30 tablets should be dispensed.

Oral Prescriptions

Prescriptions may be either written or oral. Oral prescriptions, usually received by telephone, can be received only by a pharmacist (or, in some states, a pharmacist-intern) and must be transcribed in writing immediately.

> **Note:** Always refer telephone calls from prescribers to a pharmacist.

Facsimile Prescriptions

Some state laws allow prescribers to fax prescriptions to pharmacies. Check with a pharmacist about your state's requirements.

Transferred Prescriptions

Prescription orders may be transferred from one pharmacy to another under certain circumstances. Some states require the original prescription to be cancelled. Some states do not allow prescription transfers and require that a new prescription be received from a prescriber. In most states, only pharmacists can receive or call in prescription transfers. After a pharmacist receives a transferred prescription and transcribes it onto a prescription form, a technician, in most states, may then enter the information in the computer and assist in dispensing the prescription.

INTERPRETING DIRECTIONS FOR USE

When you receive written prescriptions, the directions for use will be written by physicians in a shorthand notation sometimes referred to as a *"Sig."* (The term, "Sig.," is an abbreviation of the Latin, *Signa,* meaning "you write," which is the prescriber's instructions to put the indicated directions on the label.) Directions for use usually include: how to take the medication, how many doses to take, and when to take them.

The directions for use should include the following parts:

- Administration directions (e.g., take, insert, apply, etc.)
- Number of units in a dose and the dosage form (e.g., two tablets)
- Time or frequency of dosage (e.g., 9:00 A.M., twice daily, etc.)
- Route of administration (e.g., by mouth, on skin, etc.)

> **Note:** If the route of administration is not specified, it is usually implied by the dosage form prescribed. For example, tablets and capsules are usually taken by mouth; ointments are usually applied to the affected area of the skin, etc.

Each time you type directions for use on prescription labels, make sure you include the items mentioned above. In addition, the Sig. may sometimes contain the following:

- Length of time to continue with medication (e.g., for 10 days, until all gone, etc.)
- Reason for the medication (e.g., for pain, for high blood pressure, etc.)

Do not add information that you assume the prescriber was implying when writing the prescription without getting approval of the pharmacist. The prescriber is familiar with the patient's condition and adding directions that you assume to be correct may cause harm to the patient or inappropriate use of the medication.

Clear, accurate, and specific directions are necessary if patients are to comply with prescribers' directions. It is important that you interpret the abbreviations and directions for use accurately, so memorize the abbreviations and symbols in this section. You might try using flashcards to study the abbreviations and symbols.

Examples of Directions for Medication Administration

Medication	*Word Choice*	*Example*
Oral	Take (if an adult)	Take one (1) tablet
	Give (if a child)	Give two (2) teaspoonfuls
External	Apply	Apply to affected areas
Suppositories	Insert	Insert one (1) suppository
Drops (eye or ear)	Place or Instill	Instill one (1) drop
Inhaler (oral)	Inhale	Inhale one (1) puff

Commonly Used Abbreviations and Symbols

Number of units

a͞a	of each
ad[5]	up to
i	one
ii	two
iii	three
iv	four
v	five
x	ten; times or for
L	fifty
C	one hundred
M	one thousand
qs	as much as suffices or sufficient quantity
qs ad	add enough to make a specific quantity
s͞s	one-half
ʒ	dram or teaspoonful
℥	ounce (30 mL or 30 cc)
℥ss	1/2 ounce (one tablespoonful, 15 cc or 15 mL)

---

[5] Not to be confused with "ad" meaning "right ear."

Dosage forms

amp(s)	ampule(s)
cap(s)	capsule(s)
cr	cream
el or elix	elixir
expect	expectorant
fl	fluid
liq	liquid
lot	lotion
pulv	powder
sol	solution
supp	suppository
susp	suspension
syr	syrup
tab(s)	tablet(s)
tinc	tincture
ung or oint	ointment

Strength and systems of measurement

cc	cubic centimeter (same as mL or milliliter)
DS	double strength
ES	extra strength
fl oz	fluid ounce
g or gm	gram
gr	grain
gtt(s)	drop(s)
IU	international unit
mcg or μg	microgram
kg	kilogram
L	liter
mEq	milliequivalent
mg	milligram
mL	milliliter (same as cc or cubic centimeter)
oz	ounce
ped	pediatric strength
t or tsp	teaspoonful (ʒ , or 5 cc, or 5 mL)
T or tbsp	tablespoonful (ʒss, or 15 cc, or 15 mL)

Note: Use of the ʒ symbol as an abbreviation for teaspoon is common practice for prescribers. A fluid dram (ʒ) equals 3.69 mL and USP defines a teaspoonful as 5 mL, thus this is an example of a symbol with dual meaning and should be discouraged.

Route of administration

ad[6]	right ear
as	left ear
au	both ears or each ear
ien	in each nostril
IM	intramuscular
IV	intravenous
IVPB	intravenous piggy back
loc	locally (apply locally to affected area)
od	right eye
os	left eye
ou	both eyes or each eye
po	by mouth or orally
pr	per rectum or rectally
SC, subQ, or SQ	subcutaneous (beneath the skin)
SL	sublingual (under the tongue)
top	topically
UD or ut dict	as directed
vag	vaginal or vaginally

Time or frequency of administration

ac	before food or meals
AM	morning
ad lib	as often as needed, freely
ASAP	as soon as possible
atc	around the clock
bid	twice daily
$\overline{c}$	with daily
h, hr or °	hour, at the hour of
hs	at bedtime
noc	night
$\overline{P}$	after
pc	after food or meals
pc & hs	after meals and at bedtime
PM	in the afternoon or evening
prn	as needed
q	each or every
q4h	every four hours
qd	every day, daily
qh	every hour
qhs	every bedtime or every night at bedtime qid
	four times daily

---

[6] Not to be confused with "ad" meaning "up to" (as in "qs ad").

qod	every other day
s̄	without
stat	at once or immediately
tid	three times daily
UD or ut dict	as directed
wk	weekly

Abbreviations for controlled-release products

LA	long acting
SA	sustained action
SR	sustained release
TR	timed release

Other abbreviations

aa	affected area
ACE-I	Angiotensin Converting Enzyme Inhibitor
aff	affected
aq or aqua	water
aq dist	distilled water
ARB	Angiotensin Receptor Blocker
BC	birth control
BP	for blood pressure
COX-2	cyclooxygenase-2
cmpd	compound
DAW	dispense as written
dil	dilute
disp	dispense
DTD	give of such doses
H_2	histamine-2
H2A	Histamine-2 Antagonist
HA	for headache
HBP	for high blood pressure
MDI	Multi-dose inhaler
MDV	Multi-dose vial
NKA	no known allergies
NKDA	no known drug allergies
NR	no refills
NSAID	non-steroidal anti-inflammatory drug
PPI	proton pump inhibitor
Qty	quantity to dispense
℞	a prescription
SDV	Single-dose vial
Sig	you write (prescriber's instructions to put the indicated directions on the label)
SOB	shortness of breath
spr	spray
SSRI	serotonin-selective reuptake inhibitor

Examples of Interpreting Directions for Use

To check your learning, use the abbreviations from the groups above to interpret the following directions:

i cap tid c̄ food   Meaning: Take one (1) capsule three times a day with food.

ii gtts os qAM   Meaning: Instill two (2) drops into the left eye every morning.

> **Note:** Some pharmacists may prefer to indicate that oral medications should be taken **by mouth** even if the Sig doesn't say "po". The first example therefore would be "Take one (1) capsule by mouth three times a day with food."

Dangerous Medical Abbreviations

Many abbreviations save time and space. However, whenever abbreviations are used, there is the chance that readers will not interpret them as writers intend. The following table lists several abbreviations that should not be used, according to the Joint Commission on Accreditation of Healthcare Organizations (JCAHO).

Medical Notations	Reason to Avoid Using	Instead Use
U (unit)	Mistaken for zero, number four, or cc	Write "unit"
IU (international unit)	Mistaken for IV or number ten	Write "international unit"
QD (daily)	Mistaken for QID or QOD	Write "daily"
QOD (every other day)	Mistaken for QID and QD	Write "every other day"
Trailing zero on decimals (X.0 mg)	Decimal point is missed	Write X mg; do not include a zero after the decimal point
Lack of leading zero on decimals (.X mg)	Decimal point is missed	Write 0.X mg; use leading zero before the decimal point
MS	Can mean morphine sulfate or magnesium sulfate	Write out "morphine sulfate" or "magnesium sulfate"
MSO_4 and $MgSO_4$	Can be confused for one another	Write out "morphine sulfate" or "magnesium sulfate"

Some abbreviations are "accidents waiting to happen," so you must be especially careful in interpreting them. Even though it has been recommended that the abbreviations "qd" and "qod" not be used, you may still receive prescriptions using them. The following list contains medications that are generally administered **qd** (once a day), but never **qid** (four times a day). Try to learn them—recognizing these products will help ensure that you never confuse the two when preparing a prescription label.

Medications That Are Often Prescribed "qd" But Never "qid"

Brand Name	Generic Name
Synthroid®	levothyroxine
Lanoxin®	digoxin
Ortho-7/7/7®	ethinyl estradiol and norethindrone
Procardia® XL	nifedipine
Zyrtec®	cetirizine

Following are some examples of other potential misinterpretations:

- **"Unit"** should never be abbreviated. When the word "unit" is abbreviated as **"U"** it can be mistaken for zero, resulting in 10-fold overdoses. It is possible that the handwritten letter **"U"** could also be read as the roman numeral **"V"** or as "cc". Likewise, the abbreviation **"IU"** can be misread as **"IV"**.

- Another common error occurs with the use of the abbreviation "s̄" (for "without") has been read as "c̄," (meaning "with")."

- The abbreviation "OJ" (for "orange juice") has been misread as "OS" (for "left eye").

- The word "once" may be confused by Spanish-speaking patients as the Spanish word "*once*" (pronounced *own-say*), which is the number eleven. It is better to type out "one time."

Hints for Working with Abbreviations

- As you gain experience reading prescriptions, you will learn to read physicians' handwriting, especially those whose prescriptions you fill often.

- Become familiar with medications commonly used by particular prescribers and medications belonging to certain fields, such as ophthalmology.

- Understanding the uses of medications helps you read prescriptions more easily. For example, triazolam, taken to help patients sleep, would not be taken four times a day, but only at bedtime.

- A working knowledge of abbreviations helps interpret directions too. For example, the initials "SR," "SA," "LA," and "TR" after a medication's name tells you these are controlled-released products. These medications would not normally be taken every three to four hours or four times a day.

- Be sure to translate the directions into easily-understood terms for patients' labels. If patients do not understand directions, they cannot take their medication properly.

- If prescribers do not state the quantity of medication to dispense, you may have to calculate the quantity. For example: "i cap qid x 10 d" means "Take one capsule four times a day for 10 days." Therefore, 40 capsules should be dispensed.

Note: Never guess. If you cannot read the directions for use, or any other part of the prescription, ask a pharmacist.

Examples of Abbreviations for Medication Names

AMP	ampicillin
APAP	acetaminophen
ASA	aspirin
Ca or Ca^{++}	calcium
CDPX	chlordiazepoxide
D5W	dextrose 5% in water
DC 65	Darvon® Compound 65
DCN 100	Darvocet-N® 100
DES	diethylstilbesterol
DOSS or DSS	dioctyl sodium sulfosuccinate or docusate sodium
ECASA	enteric coated aspirin
EES	erythromycin ethylsuccinate
EPI	epinephrine
F	fluoride
FA	folic acid
Fe or Fe^{++}	iron
FeSO$_4$	ferrous sulfate
HCTZ	hydrochlorothiazide or hydrocortisone
IBU	ibuprofen
INH	Isoniazid®
K or K$^+$	potassium
KCl	potassium chloride
LR	lactated ringer's solution
MSO$_4$	morphine sulfate
MgSO$_4$	magnesium sulfate
MOM	milk of magnesia
Na or Na$^+$	sodium
NaCl	sodium chloride
NaF	sodium fluoride
NS	normal saline (0.9% sodium chloride)
NTG	nitroglycerin
PEN or PCN	penicillin
PB	phenobarbital
SMZ/TMP	sulfamethoxazole with trimethoprim
Tylenol #3	Tylenol® with Codeine 30 mg
APAP #3	acetaminophen 325 mg with codeine 30 mg
TCN	tetracycline

> **Note:** Some abbreviations for medication names are particularly dangerous, but they are still used. For example, **CPM** can be interpreted as cyclophosphamide, chlorpheniramine, chlorpromazine, or Compazine®. **PBZ** can be interpreted as phenylbutazone, pyribenzamine, or phenoxybenzamine. **HCTZ** is often used for hydrochlorothiazide but can also be used for hydrocortisone.

SELF-ASSESSMENT QUESTIONS CHAPTER IV

For each of the following prescriptions, write out the directions for use as you would put them on a prescription label:

1. 3 gtts as qid x 5 days
2. tsp qid
3. App aff area hs
4. 2 caps stat,1 tid
5. gtt ou hs
6. s̄s̄ tsp tid x 10 days
7. tab tid pc
8. 1 puff qid prn
9. supp rect prn nausea
10. 1 tab qod for heart

11. What directions should be typed on the prescription label?
    Cyclobenzaprine 10 mg tabs
    Sig: 20 mg qid x 5 days

12. A DDS may prescribe medication used to treat:
    a. Back pain.
    b. Athlete's foot.
    c. Eye infections.
    d. Toothaches.

13. All the following are required to be on a prescription except:
    a. Patient's date of birth.
    b. Patient's name.
    c. Medication name.
    d. Directions for use.

14. How should the following directions be typed on a prescription label? Sig: ii gtts ad tid UD
    a. Instill two drops in the right ear three times a day as directed.
    b. Instill two drops in the right eye three times a day as directed.
    c. Instill two drops in each eye three times a day as needed.
    d. Instill two drops in each ear three times a day as needed.

15. When written on a prescription blank, the letters "ad" stand for:
   a. As directed.
   b. Up to.
   c. Distilled water.
   d. After dinner.

16. How should the following directions be typed on a prescription label? Sig: i tab qd AM HBP
   a. Take one tablet four times each morning for high blood pressure.
   b. Take one tablet every four days in the morning for high blood pressure.
   c. Take one tablet every day in the morning for high blood pressure.
   d. Take one tablet every other morning for high blood pressure.

Answers:
1) Place (or Instill) three (3) drops into the left ear four times daily for five days.
2) Take one (1) teaspoonful four times a day.
3) Apply to the affected area at bedtime.
4) Take two (2) capsules now, then one capsule three times daily.
5) Place (or Instill) one (1) drop into each eye at bedtime.
6) Take one-half (1/2) teaspoonful three times daily for ten days.
7) Take one (1) tablet three times daily after meals.
8) Inhale one (1) puff four times daily as needed.
9) Insert one (1) suppository rectally as needed for nausea.
10) Take one (1) tablet every other day for heart.
11) Take two (2) tablets four times a day for five days. (This will be easier for the patient than saying "take 20 mg …")
12) d
13) a
14) a
15) b
16) c

Additional Practice Problems Chapter IV

Transcribe the following:

1. i tab po bid _____

2. i supp pr tid _____

3. ii caps po qd _____

4. ii cap po q4-6h _____

5. iv tabs po qhs _____

6. i cap po qid pc _____

7. i tsp po q6h _____

8. iv gtts ou qd _____

9. ii gtts as q3h _____

10. $\overline{ss}$ tsp q8h prn _____

Answers:
1. Take one (1) tablet by mouth twice daily.
2. Unwrap and insert one (1) suppository rectally three times daily.
3. Take two (2) capsules by mouth daily.
4. Take two (2) capsules by mouth every four to six hours.
5. Take four (4) tablets by mouth every night at bedtime.
6. Take one (1) capsule by mouth four times daily after meals.
7. Take (or give) one (1) teaspoonful by mouth every six hours.
8. Instill four (4) drops in each eye daily.
9. Instill two (2) drops in left ear every three hours.
10. Take (or give) one-half (1/2) teaspoonful every eight hours as needed.

Convert the following to a language patients would understand:

1. Amoxicillin 500 mg caps -1 po tid _____

2. Bactrim DS tabs – 1 po qid _____

3. Motrin 800 mg tabs -1 po qd prn _____

4. Naprosyn 375 mg tabs – 1 po bid pc _____

5. Timoptic Eye Drops – 2 gtts ou qd _____

6. Retin-A 0.1% gel – qhs x 30d ud _____

7. Lanoxin 0.125mg tabs – 1 po qam _____

8. Celebrex 100 mg caps – 2 po qpm ac _____

9. Cortisporin Otic Suspension – 3-4 gtts ad q4-6h _____

10. Cortisporin Opth Soln. - gtts 2 os q12h _____

11. Trimox 250mg/5ml susp -1tsp q8h x 14d _____

12. Lopressor 100mg tab – $\overline{ss}$ qd ud _____

13. Anucort Supp – 1 pr qhs prn _____

14. Zithromax 250mg tabs – 2 stat, 1qd x 4d _____

15. Nasalcrom – 1 spr ien 3-4 x/day _____

16. Vicodin tab – 1-2 q4-6h prn pain _____

17. Albuterol 2 mg tabs – 1 q5h atc _____

18. Voltarin Opth gtts -3 gtt ou bid x 5d _____

19. Gentamicin Opth ung -qd x 5-7d _____

Answers:
1. Take one (1) capsule by mouth three times daily.
2. Take one (1) tablet by mouth four times daily.
3. Take one (1) tablet by mouth daily as needed.
4. Take one (1) tablet by mouth twice daily after meals.
5. Instill two (2) drops in each eye daily.
6. Apply every night at bedtime for thirty days as directed.
7. Take one (1) tablet by mouth every morning.
8. Take two (2) capsules by mouth every evening before meal.
9. Instill three (3) to four (4) drops in right ear every four to six hours.
10. Instill two (2) drops in left eye every twelve hours.
11. Take (or give) one (1) teaspoonful by mouth every eight hours for fourteen days.
12. Take one-half (1/2) tablet by mouth every day as directed.
13. Unwrap and insert one (1) suppository rectally every night at bedtime as needed.
14. Take two (2) tablets by mouth immediately, then take one (1) tablet by mouth daily for four days.
15. Inhale one (1) spray in each nostril three to four times daily.
16. Take one (1) to two (2) tablets by mouth every four to six hours as needed for pain.
17. Take one (1) tablet by mouth every five hours around the clock
18. Instill three (3) drops in each eye twice daily for five days.
19. Apply ointment to affected eye(s) daily for five to seven days.

JOHN S. DOE MD
100 N. Main St.
St. Louis, MO 12345
(123) 456-7890

Name _Mike Smith_   Date _1/1/08_

Address _1234 State St._

Protonix 40 mg   #60
Take 1 tab PO BID

Refills _1 (one)_

DEA # _____

_____ _Doe_ _____
Dispense as written   Substitution permitted

Prescription #1

1. This prescription was written for Protonix. If the medication is taken as prescribed, everyday, how many days will this prescription last?

JOHN S. DOE MD
100 N. Main St.
St. Louis, MO 12345
(123) 456-7890

Name _Mike Smith_   Date _1/1/08_

Address _1234 State St._

Atrovent Inhaler #1 2-3 puff TID
Flovent 110 mcg #1 2-3 puff BID

Refills _5 (five)_

DEA # _____

_____ _Doe_ _____
Dispense as written   Substitution permitted

Prescription #2

1. By reading the box for the Atrovent Inhaler, you find that each inhaler contains 200 inhalations. What is the days' supply that should be entered into the computer for the Atrovent prescription?

2. Flovent is dispensed in a 13 g canister that contains 120 metered doses. What is the days' supply that should be entered into the computer for the Flovent prescription?

Answers:
Prescription # 1:
1)   30 days

Prescription # 2:
1)   22 days
2)   20 days

John S. Doe MD
100 N. Main St.
St. Louis, MO 12345
(123) 456-7890

Name _*Jane Smith*_   Date _1/1/08_

Address _1234 State St._

Ortho-Novum 777 28 day
Take 1 tab PO daily

Refills _6 (six)_

DEA # _____

_____ _Doe_ _____
Dispense as written   Substitution permitted

Prescription # 3

1. What is the total number of compacts indicated by this prescription?

John S. Doe MD
100 N. Main St.
St. Louis, MO 12345
(123) 456-7890

Name _*Jane Smith*_   Date _1/1/08_

Address _1234 State St._

Bactrim DS 20
Take 1 tab PO BID

Refills _0 (zero)_

DEA # _____

_____ _Doe_ _____
Dispense as written   Substitution permitted

Prescription # 4

1. As you are entering this prescription in the computer, an allergy warning is displayed on the computer screen. What type of allergy does Jane Smith have?

Answers:
Prescription # 3:
1)   7 compacts

Prescription # 4:
1) Sulfa drugs

John S. Doe MD
100 N. Main St.
St. Louis, MO 12345
(123) 456-7890

Name _Jane Smith_   Date _1/1/08_

Address _1234 State St._

Lorabid 200 mg/ 5ml

i ʒ PO BID x 10

Refills _0 (zero)_

DEA # _____

_____ _Doe_ _____
Dispense as written   Substitution permitted

John S. Doe MD
100 N. Main St.
St. Louis, MO 12345
(123) 456-7890

Name _Jane Smith_   Date _1/1/08_

Address _1234 State St._

Amoxicillin 500 mg 2 PO BID x 7

Biaxin 500 mg PO BID x 7

Aciphex 20 mg PO BID x 7

Refills _0 (zero)_

DEA # _____

_____ _Doe_ _____
Dispense as written   Substitution permitted

Prescription # 5

1. What directions should be placed on the label for this prescription?

Prescription # 6

1. How many capsules should be dispensed for the amoxicillin?
2. How many tablets should be dispensed for the Aciphex?

Answers:
Prescription # 5:
1) Take (or Give) one (1) teaspoonful by mouth twice daily for 10 days.
Prescription # 6:
1) 28 capsules
2) 14 tablets

PHARMACY TECHNICIAN COMPETENCY ASSESSMENT

CHAPTER IV

Description of Ability or Skill	Initials		Training Completed	
	Tech	R.Ph.	Date	Remarks
The technician trainee understands and can cite examples of those persons who may prescribe medications.				
The technician trainee understands and can cite the information required on completed prescription forms.				
The technician trainee can identify and interpret the various methods used to indicate the quantity of medication to dispense.				
The technician trainee is able to correctly translate a prescriber's directions for use into accurate and complete directions for the patient.				
The technician trainee is familiar with the ways in which abbreviations can be misinterpreted.				

Chapter V
Pharmacy Calculations
By: Steven M. Gullette and Kenneth W. Schafermeyer

EDUCATIONAL OBJECTIVES

After studying the material in this chapter, the technician trainee should be able to:

- Use the four systems of measurement used in pharmacies and be able to convert from one to another
- Use Roman numerals
- Calculate ratios and proportions
- Calculate dilutions of stock solutions
- Calculate percentage preparations (i.e., w/w, w/v, v/v)
- Calculate IV flow rates and infusion time
- Convert Celsius to Fahrenheit and from Fahrenheit to Celsius
- Calculate prescription dosages, quantities and days supply
- Calculate children's dosages
- Perform basic business calculations (e.g., gross margin, mark-up, and inventory turnover)

SYSTEMS OF MEASUREMENT

As a pharmacy technician, you must calculate accurately and convert between different systems of measurement. Pharmacy uses four interrelated systems:

- Metric system
- Apothecary system
- Avoirdupois system
- Common household measures

Since you will need to be familiar with a number of conversions between these measurement systems, try to memorize the information provided below.

Metric system. All stock bottles of prescription medications include a metric weight or volume on the package label. Some products are also measured in one of the other systems. Weights and measures in the metric system are the easiest to work with because they are based on units of ten.

- Weight in the metric system. The gram, (g or gm) is the base unit. There are 1,000 milligrams (mg) in one gram and 1,000 grams in one kilogram (kg). There are about 30 gm in 1 ounce.

Note: For the metric system use decimals—not fractions. For example, do not write 1/2 gm; write 0.5 gm (or 500 mg) instead.

- **Liquids in the metric system.** When measuring liquids in the metric system, the base unit is the liter (l or L). There are 1,000 milliliters (mL) in one liter; the prefix, *milli,* means "one thousandth." Sometimes you will see dosages written in cubic centimeters (cc). This unit has the same value as, and is therefore interchangeable with, milliliters for liquids.

It is useful to remember that 30 mL equals one fluid ounce (fl oz). Therefore, a four-ounce bottle of medication contains 120 mL. A liter is slightly larger than a quart, a unit of the household system.

Metric Weight and Volume

Weight

1 kilogram (kg)	=	1,000 gm
1 milligram (mg)	=	0.001 gm or 1,000 mcg
1 microgram (μg or mcg)	=	0.001 mg
1 gram (gm)	=	1,000 mg

Volume

1 milliliter (mL)	=	0.001 liter
1 liter (L)	=	1,000 mL

Apothecary system. This system is old and awkward. Nevertheless, because of tradition, we still see products labeled in the apothecary system and some physicians still write prescriptions using apothecary notations.

- **Weight in the apothecary system.** The standard for measuring weight in this system is a grain (gr). This standard was devised in ancient times based on the average weight of a grain of wheat. To give you a reference, the active ingredient in a regular-strength aspirin tablet weighs slightly more than five grains. (The additional weight of inactive ingredients is not included; therefore the tablet itself weighs more than five grains.)

Very few products are still measured in grains. Some patients continue to ask for five-grain aspirin. In this situation, you need to know that 5 gr = 325 mg. The common dosage for this product is 10 gr (650 mg), or two tablets. Stock bottles from which you dispense medication will include the product's strength in the metric system.

- **Liquids in the apothecary system.** The unit of volume is the fluid dram. One fluid dram is approximately equal to five mL (five cc) in metric units and one teaspoonful in the household system. A fluid dram is abbreviated "fl dr" and is often represented by the symbol "ʒ."

Apothecary Weight and Volume

Weight

60 grains (gr)	=	1 dram (dr. or ʒ)
8 drams (dr)	=	1 ounce (℥)

Volume

8 fluid drams (ʒ viii)	=	1 fluid ounce (fl oz or ℥ i)
16 fluid ounces	=	1 pint (pt)
2 pints	=	1 quart (qt)
4 quarts	=	1 gallon (gal)

Avoirdupois system. The avoirdupois system is used in commerce by manufacturers and suppliers of medications, chemicals and other materials by weight. Pharmacists who purchase bulk or prepackaged amounts of medications or chemicals purchase them in the avoirdupois system. Sixteen avoirdupois ounces (oz) are equal to 1 pound (lb).

Common household measures. When patients measure a dose of liquid medication at home, they usually use a teaspoon. For this reason, most liquid dosages are formulated to contain the medication a person needs in one teaspoonful (tsp) or, occasionally, in a multiple of teaspoonfuls. Household teaspoonfuls can vary, however, from three mL to seven mL. Therefore, pharmacists often recommend that patients use a one-teaspoon (5 mL) measuring spoon or purchase a dosing spoon from the pharmacy department.

A few liquid medications requiring larger doses, such as antacids, are given in tablespoonfuls (tbsp). The tablespoon holds approximately 15 mL or about one-half fluid ounce.

Most liquid medications supplied to pharmacies come in pint (or sometimes one-gallon) containers. One pint equals 16 fl oz. You learned earlier that there are approximately 30 mL in 1 fl oz. Therefore, there are approximately 480 mL in one pint.

Note: Do not be alarmed if you look at the label on a one-pint bottle and see that it contains 473 mL. The reason for this is that there are actually 29.57 mL in a fluid ounce. However, for the sake of convenience, you may round the figure to 30 mL per fluid oz.

Most over-the-counter (OTC) medications carry both metric and household notations. For example, the label on a bottle of Robitussin® (the brand name for a cough medication) tells you that each teaspoonful (5 mL) contains 100 mg of guaifenesin (the active ingredient).

Here are some important equivalents for you to know. You might want to use flashcards to help you memorize them.

Common Household Measures	
Household Measure	**Approximate Metric Equivalent**
one-half teaspoonful (ʒ ss̄)	2.5 mL
one teaspoonful (ʒ i)	5 mL
two teaspoonfuls (ʒ ii)	10 mL
three teaspoonfuls = 1 tablespoonful =	
one-half ounce (℥ ss̄)	15 mL
two tablespoonfuls	30 mL

As a pharmacy technician, you will frequently calculate how much medication you should dispense so that it will last the required number of days. For practice, calculate the amount of Amoxicillin you would need to fill this prescription:

Amoxicillin 250 mg/5 mL

Sig: ʒ i tid x 10 days

By reading the prescription, you know that:

Dosage = ʒ i = 5 mL
Frequency = tid = 3 times a day
Duration = 10 days

So the order "ʒ i tid x 10 days" calls for 5 mL three times a day, for 10 days.

Therefore, you would need 150 mL of Amoxicillin (5 mL x 3 times a day x 10 days).

Intersystem Conversion

It is sometimes advantageous to convert the weight or fluid volume from one system to another. Following is a table of those equivalents commonly used in pharmacy. Usually the approximate metric equivalent listed in the middle column is sufficient.

Conversion Equivalents of Weight

(Apothecary or Avoirdupois) Measure	Approximate Metric Equivalent	Exact Metric Equivalent
1 grain (gr)	60 mg	64.8 mg
1/2 grain	30 mg	32.4 mg
1/4 grain	15 mg	16.2 mg
1/60 grain	1 mg	1.08 mg
1/100 grain	0.6 mg (600 mcg)	0.648 mg
1/150 grain	0.4 mg (400 mcg)	0.432 mg
1/200 grain	0.3 mg (300 mcg)	0.324 mg
1/300 grain	0.2 mg (200 mcg)	0.216 mg
1/400 grain	0.15 mg (150 mcg)	0.162 mg
1 ounce avoir (oz)	30 gm	28.35 gm
16 oz avoir (1 pound or 1 lb)	480 gm	454 gm
2.2 pounds avoir		1,000 gm (1 kg)

Conversion Equivalents of Volume

Apothecary Measure	Approximate Metric Equivalent	Exact Metric Equivalent
1 fluid ounce (1 fl ʒ)	30 mL	29.57 mL
4 fluid ounces	120 mL	118.28 mL
8 fluid ounces	240 mL	236.56 mL
16 fluid ounces (1 pint)	480 mL	473 mL
2 pints (1 quart)	960 mL	946 mL
4 quarts (1 gallon)	3,840 mL	3,784 mL

ROMAN NUMERALS

Understanding Roman numerals is essential to accurately read and fill prescriptions. Roman numerals are commonly used on prescriptions to designate strength or quantity, the number of doses and the amount of a drug in the directions. Also, the DEA uses Roman numerals to signify scheduling of controlled substances (see Chapter III). The directions for use must be relayed to patients in a way that is easy for them to understand.

Converting Roman to Arabic numbers. Prescriptions may contain a combination of Roman and Arabic numerals. The following is a list of the most common values.

s̄s̄	=	½	L or l	=	50
I or i	=	1	C or c	=	100
V or v	=	5	D or d	=	500
X or x	=	10	M or m	=	1000

Rules for using Roman numerals. The two main differences between Roman and Arabic numbers are that Roman numerals lack a character for the number zero and character placement can indicate subtraction or addition. Rules for working with Roman numerals and examples are shown below.

- When a letter is repeated, its value is repeated (e.g., XXX = 10 + 10 + 10 = 30).
- A letter cannot be repeated more than three times (e.g., IIII is not equal to 4).
- V, L, D can never be repeated, and are never subtracted from larger numbers; VV is not equal to 10 and VL is not equal to 45.
- When a smaller number is placed in front of a larger one, it is subtracted (e.g., CM = 900).
- When an equal or smaller number is placed after the larger number, it is added (e.g., XI = 11).
- You can never subtract more than one numeral; IIX is not equal to 8.

RATIO AND PROPORTION

One of the most important calculations concepts for pharmacy technicians is ratio and proportion. A ratio is the relationship between two quantities. For example, the ratio of a to b is shown as: $\frac{a}{b}$ or a:b

A common situation in pharmacy is the drug concentration to solution. If there are 5 g of Dextrose in 100 mL of water, this is expressed as: $\frac{5 \text{ g}}{100 \text{ mL}}$

A proportion is the equal relationship between two ratios. For example, the proportion of a to b and c to d is expressed as: $\frac{a}{b} = \frac{c}{d}$ or a:b = c:d

Using the previous drug concentration example, we can say that $\frac{5 \text{ g}}{100 \text{ mL}} = \frac{50 \text{ g}}{1000 \text{ mL}}$

The numerators can be divided into their denominators twenty times which makes the ratios equivalent. Another way to show that the ratios are equivalent is by cross-multiplication. The numerator of the first ratio (a) times the denominator of the second ratio (d) equals the numerator of the second ratio (c) times the denominator of the first ratio (b). You need to move terms from one side of the equation to the other by cancellation of equal values. This can be represented by:

$(\cancel{100 \text{ mL}}) \dfrac{5 \text{ g}}{\cancel{100 \text{ mL}}} = \dfrac{50 \text{ g}}{1000 \text{ mL}} \text{ x } 100 \text{ mL}$ **multiply both sides by 100 mL and cancel equal terms and units**

$5 \text{ g x } 1000 \text{ mL} = (\cancel{1000 \text{ mL}}) \dfrac{50 \text{ g}}{\cancel{1000 \text{ mL}}} \text{ x } 100 \text{ mL}$

$5 \text{ g x } 1000 \text{ mL} = 50 \text{ g x } 100 \text{ mL}$

$5000 = 5000$

Mathematical problems are made up of known and unknown terms. Oftentimes, the value of one term is unknown. An unknown term is called a variable, generally represented by the letter x. In this situation, you would substitute x for the unknown and cross-multiply as above, solving for x. The equation is then written as:

$$\frac{x}{b} = \frac{c}{d}$$

Next, multiply both sides by b to determine the value of x.

$$(\cancel{b}) \frac{x}{\cancel{b}} = \frac{c}{d} \text{ x } b$$

$$x = \frac{cb}{d}$$

Therefore, the above concentration equation can be solved for an unknown when written as:

$$\frac{x}{100 \text{ mL}} = \frac{50 \text{ g}}{1000 \text{ mL}}$$

multiply both sides by 100 mL and cancel equal terms and solve for x

$$(\cancel{100 \text{ mL}})\frac{x}{\cancel{100 \text{ mL}}} = \frac{50 \text{ g}}{1000 \cancel{\text{ mL}}} \text{ x } 100 \cancel{\text{ mL}}$$

$$X = \frac{5000 \text{ g}}{1000}$$

solve for x

$$x = 5 \text{ g}$$

Rules for solving ratio-proportion problems. In order to solve ratio-proportion problems, there are two important rules. Three of the four terms must be known and the units on each side of the equation must be kept in the same order (e.g., g/mL = g/mL).

Ratio-proportion problems are not only seen when determining drug concentration / solution. These equations are frequently used when prescriptions call for tablets or capsules to be taken by a patient according to a regimen. Consider the following situations:

A prescription is written for Atenolol 25 mg po BID x 30 days. How many tablets are required to fill this prescription?

What is known?	2 tablets / day
What is unknown?	total number of tablets needed in 30 days
What is the unknown ratio?	x tablets / 30 days

Step 1: Place the known ratio on the right side of the equation

$$\frac{x}{30 \text{ days}} = \frac{2 \text{ tablets}}{1 \text{ day}}$$

Step 2: Cross-multiply to get x alone on one side

$$(\cancel{30 \text{ days}})\frac{x}{\cancel{30 \text{ days}}} = \frac{2 \text{ tablets}}{\cancel{1 \text{ day}}} \text{ x } 30 \cancel{\text{ days}}$$

Step 3: Solve for x

$$x = 60 \text{ tablets}$$

SPECIFIC GRAVITY

Specific gravity is the density of a substance in relation to the density of water. Because water is what all other substances are compared to, water has a specific gravity of 1.00 or a density of 1.00 g/mL. Specific gravity and density can be thought as the thickness of a solution or substance. We would expect pancake syrup to have a higher specific gravity than orange juice or milk because pancake syrup tends to be thicker than orange juice or milk.

The difference between specific gravity and density is that specific gravity is a direct comparison of the density of a substance to the density of water; therefore specific gravity has no units. Density is simply the mass of substance contained in the volume of the substance. For our purposes the two are identical except specific gravity has no units and density has units in "g/mL."

While technicians seldom calculate specific gravity problems, an understanding of specific gravity and density is useful in calculating percent weight-weight (%w/w), percent weight-volume (%w/v), and percent volume-volume (%v/v) problems and converting among these measures.

Examples:

7 grams of substance A is dissolved in 100 mL of solution B.
The density of solution B is 1.205 g/mL.
The density of substance A is 1.86 g/mL.
Calculate %w/w, %w/v, and %v/v.

Percent weight-weight (%w/w) in this problem is the grams of substance A divided by the grams in solution B multiplied by 100. The density of solution B is used to convert 100 mL of B into grams of B.

$$\frac{7 \text{ g A}}{100 \text{ mL B}} \times \frac{1 \text{ mL B}}{1.205 \text{ g B}} \times 100 = 5.8\% \text{ (w/w)}$$

Percent weight-volume (%w/v) in this problem is the grams of substance A divided by the mL of solution B multiplied by 100. The density does not have to be used because the values needed are already given.

$$\frac{7 \text{ g A}}{100 \text{ mL B}} \times 100 = 7\% \text{ (w/v)}$$

Percent volume-volume (%v/v) in this problem is the mL of substance A divided by the mL of solution B multiplied by 100. The density of substance A is used to convert 7 grams of substance A into mL of substance A.

$$\frac{7 \text{ g A}}{100 \text{ mL B}} \times \frac{1 \text{ mL A}}{1.86 \text{ g A}} \times 100 = 3.8\% \text{ (v/v)}$$

TONICITY

Tonicity is the osmotic pressure of a solution. Osmotic pressure is the pressure, usually due to salt concentration, that is required to prevent osmosis, or the movement of water across a membrane. And because water moves in attempt to equalize the concentrations, tonicity is important when administering several dosage forms such as parenterals and eye drops. These types of dosage forms must be "isotonic," which means that they must have the same tonicity or osmotic pressure as the body fluid where the drug is administered.

For example, IVs, TPNs, and injections are all administered into the blood stream. If an IV is hypertonic (having a higher osmotic pressure or salt concentration than the blood) osmosis will result in the movement of water out of the red blood cells. The movement of water out of red blood cells causes the cells to shrivel resulting in decreased oxygen carried to organs and tissues. On the other hand, if an IV is hypotonic (having a lower osmotic pressure or salt concentration than the blood), then water moves into red blood cells. The movement of water into red blood cells causes the cells to burst (hemolyze) also resulting in decreased oxygen carried to organs and tissues.

Therefore, making sure that IVs and injections are isotonic is crucial. Solutions are made isotonic by adding salt (also known as "sodium chloride" and abbreviated "NaCl"). The osmotic pressure of the blood is 0.9% (or 0.9 g of sodium chloride in 100 mL of blood) so solutions must also be 0.9%(w/v) when administered into the blood stream. Normal saline IVs are 0.9% NaCl and are often used to administer IV medications. If purified water is used instead of normal saline, the tonicity of the solution must be adjusted so that it is isotonic. Look at the following tonicity problem:

How much sodium chloride (NaCl) is required to make a 70 mL solution isotonic?
Normal osmotic pressure of the blood is 0.9% NaCl; therefore the following proportion can be used:

$$\frac{0.9 \text{ g}}{100 \text{ mL}} = \frac{? \text{ g}}{70 \text{ mL}}$$

70 mL x 0.9 g = 100mL x ?g
63 = 100mL x ?g
$\frac{63}{100}$ = 0.63 g

0.63 grams of sodium chloride is needed to make the solution isotonic. Some products may appear to not have enough NaCl in them. This is because ingredients already have an NaCl equivalent. For example, a preparation includes ingredients A, B, and NaCl, and 0.63 grams of NaCl are required to make the solution isotonic. If ingredient A has a NaCl equivalent of 0.03 g and ingredient B has a NaCl equivalent of 0.1 g, then the solution would only need 0.5 g of NaCl because 0.13 g of NaCl are contained in the ingredients.

DILUTION OF STOCK SOLUTIONS

You may be asked to change the concentration of prepared stock solutions, ointments or creams according to a prescriber's instructions. This is accomplished using the following formula:

$$(C1) \times (V1) = (C2) \times (V2)$$

C1 = the concentration or strength of the stock product
V1 = the weight or volume of the stock product
C2 = the concentration or strength of the desired product
V2 = the weight or volume of the desired product

Again you need to organize the equation using the known terms on the right and the unknown term (x) on the left. For example, you have 0.9% normal saline (NS) solution but a prescription calls for 250 mL of ½ NS. This equation can be stated as:

$$(0.9\%) \times (x \text{ mL}) = (0.45\%) \times (250\text{mL}) \qquad \textbf{since 0.45\% is half of 0.9\%}$$
$$x = 125\text{mL of } 0.9\%\text{NS}$$

The next step determines how much water you should add to the 0.9% stock solution to make the desired solution which is shown by:

$$(\text{Final volume}) - (\text{stock volume}) = \text{volume of water}$$
$$(250 \text{ mL}) - (125 \text{ mL}) = 125 \text{ mL of water}$$

Therefore, you would take 125 mL of the 0.9%NS and add 125 mL water for a final concentration of 0.45%NS.

The Alligation Method. Another way to prepare a product of a desired strength is by mixing stronger and weaker solids or solutions. The amounts of the ingredients can be determined by using the alligation alternate. This is a weighted average of the components, meaning that the desired product strength must lie somewhere in between the weaker and stronger strength components. The number of parts of each component can be found by using a simple schematic as demonstrated below.

Strength available	Desired strength	Parts needed
a		x
	c	
b		y

a = the higher concentration
b = the lower concentration
c = the desired concentration

x = parts of the higher concentration needed
y = parts of the lower concentration needed

We can find the number of parts needed once we have entered the information for the terms a, b and c. This is shown by the equation:

$$\frac{x}{y} = \frac{c - b}{a - c}$$

For example, how many mL of 3% Acetic Acid must be mixed with 15% Acetic acid to give 2500 mL of 10% Acetic Acid?

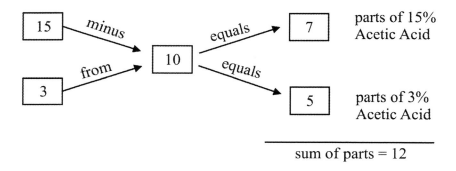

There are 12 total parts of the 2500 mL mixture. Set up a ratio to find the amount of 15% Acetic Acid to use. Then, subtract that amount from 2500 mL to find the amount of 3 % Acetic Acid to use.

$$\frac{12}{2500} = \frac{7}{x}$$

$$12x = 7\,(2500)$$

$$12x = 17,500$$

$$x = 1458 \text{ mL of 15\% Acetic Acid}$$

$$2500 \text{ mL} - 1458 \text{ mL} = 1042 \text{ mL of 3\% Acetic Acid}$$

Percentage. The unknown "parts" of each ingredient used can be found using another method, as well. Using the previous problem (how many mL of 3% Acetic Acid must be mixed with 15% Acetic acid to give 2500 mL of 10% Acetic Acid?), we can set up the equation:

$$ax + by = c\,(x + y)$$

a = Percent of Higher Concentration
b = Percent of Lower Concentration
c = Percent of Resulting Concentration
x = Parts of A (Parts of Higher Concentration)
y = Parts of B (Parts of Lower Concentration)
x + y = Parts of Resulting Concentration

Step 1: Establish values for the terms

$$a = 15\%$$
$$b = 3\%$$
$$c = 10\%$$
$$x + y = 2500\text{mL}$$

Step 2: Solve for x

$$ax + by = c\,(x + y)$$

$$15x + 3\,(2500 - x) = 10\,(2500\text{mL})$$

$$15x + 7500 - 3x = 25000$$

$$12x = 17500$$

$$x = 1458$$

- Remember x = mL for 15% and Y = mL for 3%
- Since x = 1458 mL, we need 1458 mL of 15% Acetic Acid

Step 3: Solve for y

$$x + y = 2500 \text{ mL}$$

$$x = 1458 \text{ mL}$$

$$2500 - 1458 = 1042$$

$$y = 1042 \text{ mL of 3% Acetic Acid}$$

PERCENTAGE PREPARATIONS

Percent (%) means "in a hundred." Percentage is used to express the concentration of active and inactive components in a solid or liquid. Pharmaceutical preparations are characterized as followed:

- Percent weight-in-volume (%w/v) means the number of grams of an ingredient in 100 mL of liquid.
- Percent weight-in weight (%w/w) means the number of grams of an ingredient in 100 g of solid or semi-solid.
- Percent volume-in-volume (%v/v) means the number of milliliters of an ingredient in 100 mL of a liquid.

The percentage strength of a preparation is generally calculated by setting up a proportion equation. For example, if you want to know how much Dextrose is in a 1 L bag of Dextrose 5% in Water (D5W), since 5 % dextrose means that there are 5 grams of dextrose in 100 mL, you would set up the following equation:

$$\frac{x \text{ g}}{1000 \text{ mL}} = \frac{5 \text{ g}}{100 \text{ mL}}$$

$$(\cancel{1000}) \frac{x \text{ g}}{\cancel{1000} \text{ mL}} = \frac{5 \text{ g} \times 1000 \cancel{\text{ mL}}}{100 \cancel{\text{ mL}}}$$

$$x = 50 \text{ g}$$

FLOW RATE CALCULATIONS

Flow rate provides information on the volume of fluid or amount of drug a patient will receive over a period of time. The solution may be given by injection, considering it's a small amount, and administered by the nursing staff via needle and syringe. When an IV fluid is hung next to the patient's bed, the fluid can either drip into the vein via gravity or by electric infusion pump. The units for flow rate calculations are mL/hr or, if calculating for a pump, the units are mL/min. Ratio and proportion calculations are used to determine the variables and ratios for flow rate equations. A physician will specify the amount of fluid and the duration of time that it should be infused based upon a patient's requirements. It is then up to the pharmacist or pharmacy technician to calculate the number of drops per minute or drops per hour needed to fulfill the order.

For example, you receive a prescription written for 10 mEq KCl and 10 mEq K Acetate in 1000 mL D5W ordered by a physician to be administered over 6 hours. What is the rate in mL/min? What is the rate in mL/hour?

$$x = ML$$

$$\frac{x \, mL}{1 \, min} = \frac{1000 \, mL}{360 \, min}$$

$$x = \frac{(1 \, \cancel{min}) \, 1000 \, mL}{360 \, \cancel{min}}$$

$$x = 2.8 \, mL/min$$

$$\frac{2.8 \, mL \, x \, (60 \, \cancel{min})}{1 \, \cancel{min} \quad 1 \, hr} = 168 \, mL/hr$$

If you receive an order to infuse 1000 mL D5W over 12 hours via an infusion pump and the tube set dispenses 10 drops/mL, the following formula is used to calculate a flow rate:

$$Drops / minute = \frac{mL \ of \ solution \ x \ \# \ of \ drops/mL}{minutes \ of \ administration \ (hrs \ x \ 60)}$$

$$gtts/min = \frac{1000 \ x \ 10}{12 \ x \ 60}$$

$$gtts/min = 14$$

Note: Infusion sets can deliver milliliters in a specific number of drops. It is important to know the infusion set size that will be used in order to know the number of drops/mL that will be delivered.

INFUSION TIME CALCULATIONS

Infusion time calculations are similar to flow-rate calculations. In this case, we want to know the amount of time that it will take for a specified amount of solution to be administered to the patient. The following equation should be used:

Total volume of infusion x drops x minutes x 1 hr
                                    mL   drops   60 min

Example: What time interval will be needed for the administration of 1000 mL D5W if an infusion set delivers 10 drops/mL and is set at 20 drops/min?

1000 ~~mL~~ x 10 ~~drops~~ x 1 ~~min~~ x 1 hr = 8.3 hours
                ~~mL~~   20 ~~drops~~ 60 ~~min~~

TEMPERATURE

Temperature conversion. It is important to understand the Fahrenheit and Celsius scales to measure temperature since both are commonly used in pharmacy practice. The freezing and boiling points of water on the Celsius ($^\circ$ C) scale are 0° and 100°, respectively. On the Fahrenheit ($^\circ$ F) scale the freezing and boiling points are 32° and 212°, respectively. One formula is used in order to convert between the two:

$$9 \times {}^\circ C = (5 \times {}^\circ F) - 160$$

Example: Convert 15 degrees Celsius to Fahrenheit

$$9 \times 15 = 5F - 160$$

$$135 = 5F - 160$$
$$\underline{+\,160 = +\,160}$$
$$295 = 5F$$

$$\frac{295}{5} = \frac{5F}{5}$$

$$F = 59$$

Example: Convert 70 degrees Fahrenheit to Celsius

$$9 \times C = (5 \times 70) - 160$$

$$9C = 190$$

$$\frac{9C}{9} = \frac{190}{9}$$

$$C = 21.1$$

DRUG DOSAGE CALCULATIONS

Drug dosage based on age. Drug dose based on age is an extremely inaccurate tool for determination of a dose. One should not determine drug dosage based on age if other data, such as body weight, is available to calculate the dose.

Drug dosage based on body weight. In most medical guidelines, the dose of a particular drug is given in terms of "mg of drug per kg of body weight." This allows for flexibility of individual dose calculation based on patient's weight.

Example: If the package insert of Chlorambucil indicated a normal dose for Chlorambucil to be 150µg/kg of body weight once daily and we have a patient who weighs 154 lbs, we can easily calculate their dose.

First, convert lbs to kg (1 kg = 2.2 lbs):

$$\frac{x \text{ kg}}{154 \text{ lbs}} = \frac{1 \text{ kg}}{2.2 \text{ lbs}}$$

$$x = 70 \text{ kg}$$

Then calculate the dose:

$$\frac{x \mu g}{70 \text{ kg}} = \frac{150 \mu g}{1 \text{ kg}}$$

$$X = 10,500 \mu g \text{ (or 10.5 mg)}$$

Children's dosing. Since drug dosages in many reference books are given for adults, there are several formulas that can be used to determine the dose of a drug for a child. A quick formula known as Clark's Rule follows this equation:

$$\frac{\text{weight of child (lbs)} \times \text{adult dose}}{150} = \text{child's dose}$$

Example: If an adult dose is 30 drops once per day, what is the dose for a 50 lb child?

$$\frac{50}{150} \times 30 \text{ drops} = \text{child's dose}$$

$$\frac{1}{3} \times 30 \text{ drops} = 10 \text{ drops once per day}$$

Using Clark's Rule does not take other factors into account such as height, age, etc. A more accurate equation for determining children's dosages is the Body Surface Area (BSA) formula. Pharmacies have charts known as "nomograms" to help you find body surface area based on the patient's weight and height. A line is drawn between the three columns of the chart and the BSA, given in square meters, is interpreted from the intersection. The child's BSA is entered into the equation divided by 1.73 m^2 which is the average adult BSA. That term is multiplied by the average adult dose given in the reference source. The equation is stated as:

$$\frac{\text{child's BSA}}{1.73} \times \text{adult dose} = \text{child's dose}$$

Example: If an adult dose is 30 drops once per day, what is the dose for a child with a BSA of 0.6 m^2?

$$\frac{0.6}{1.73} \times 30 \text{ drops} = \text{child's dose}$$

$$0.35 \times 30 \text{ drops} = 10 \text{ drops once per day}$$

MILLIEQUIVALENTS

Milliequivalent (mEq) is the unit of measure for electrolytes in solution and are often used in hospitals. Electrolytes are substances which conduct an electrical current and are found in the body's blood, tissue fluids, and cells. The formula for expression of a milliequivalent concentration is determined by the ratio of atomic weight to valence – general chemistry topics that are beyond the scope of this Manual. For more detailed information, see your pharmacist.

Salts & saline solution are examples of electrolyte solutions. Other examples include:

- $NaCl$ (sodium chloride)
- $MgSO_4$ (magnesium sulfate)
- KCl (potassium chloride)
- K Acetate   (potassium acetate)
- Ca Gluconate   (calcium gluconate)
- Na Acetate   (sodium acetate)

Electrolytes are added to TPN (total parenteral nutrition) orders specified by the physician dependent upon a patient's condition. The pharmacy technician will generally calculate the amount of each electrolyte needed and add the amounts requested to the solution. Again, ratio and proportion and percent solution equations will be used to determine the amounts needed. After the ingredients are added, the vials and calculation sheets are saved and displayed for the pharmacist to perform a final check.

Example: You are asked to make a TPN order as follows. The total volume is to equal 1000 mL. What amount of each ingredient is required to make the order?

TPN Order	Material available in your pharmacy	
Aminosyn 4.25%	Aminosyn 8.5%	1000mL
Dextrose 25%	Dextrose 70%	1000mL
Additives:		
NaCl 24 mEq	NaCl 4.4 mEq/mL	20mL vial
KCl 22 mEq	KCl 2mEq/mL	20mL vial
MVI (multi-vitamin)10mL	MVI	10mL vial
Sterile Water (qs ad)		

Aminosyn:

$0.0425 \times 1000 \text{ mL} = 42.5 \text{ g needed}$

$$\frac{x \text{ mL}}{42.5 \text{ g}} = \frac{100 \text{ mL}}{8.5 \text{ g}}$$

$$\frac{(42.5 \text{ g}) \, x \text{ mL}}{42.5 \text{ g}} = \frac{100 \text{ mL}}{8.5 \text{ g}} \times 42.5 \text{ g}$$

$$x = 500 \text{ mL}$$

Dextrose:

$0.25 \times 1000 \text{ mL} = 250 \text{ g needed}$

$$\frac{x \text{ mL}}{250 \text{ g}} = \frac{100 \text{ mL}}{70 \text{ g}}$$

$$\frac{(250 \text{ g}) \, x \text{ mL}}{250 \text{ g}} = \frac{100 \text{ mL}}{70 \text{ g}} \times 250 \text{g}$$

$$x = 357 \text{ mL}$$

NaCl:

$$\frac{x \text{ mL}}{24 \text{ mEq}} = \frac{1 \text{ mL}}{4.4 \text{ mEq}}$$

$$\frac{(24 \text{mEq}) \, x \text{ mL}}{24 \text{ mEq}} = \frac{1 \text{ mL}}{4.4 \text{ mEq}} \times 24 \text{ mEq}$$

$$X = 5.45 \text{ mL}$$

KCl:

$$\frac{x \text{ mL}}{22 \text{ mEq}} = \frac{1 \text{ mL}}{2 \text{ mEq}}$$

$$\frac{(22 \text{ mEq}) \, x \text{ mL}}{22 \text{ mEq}} = \frac{1 \text{ mL}}{2 \text{ mEq}} \times 22 \text{ mEq}$$

$$x = 11 \text{ mL}$$

MVI: Add the 10 mL of multi-vitamin

Sterile Water: Add enough sterile water to make 1000 mL after all other quantities have been subtracted from the total volume.

Sterile water needed =		1000 mL
	minus	500 mL
	minus	357 mL
	minus	5.45 mL
	minus	11 mL
	minus	10 mL
	equals	116.55 mL sterile water

BUSINESS CALCULATIONS

Gross margin (GM). The gross margin (also known as "gross profit") can be calculated for all sales over a period of time or for the sale of an individual item.

For all sales over a period of time, the GM is calculated as the difference between sales and the pharmacy's cost of the merchandise sold (known as "cost of goods sold" or "COGS")

For the sale of an individual item the GM is difference between a product's selling price and the pharmacy's acquisition cost for the product that was sold (also referred to as COGS). Gross margin can be calculated as a dollar amount or as a percentage of the selling price.

GM in dollars = Selling price – COGS

GM as a % of sales = (Selling price – COGS) ÷ Selling price

= GM (in dollars) ÷ Selling price

Mark-up. The difference between the acquisition cost and the selling price is the mark-up. The mark-up, therefore, is the same as the gross margin.

Mark-up = Selling price – COGS

Mark-up is usually calculated as a percentage. Sometimes it is calculated as a percentage of cost; more commonly, it is calculated as a percentage of the selling price (i.e., the same as the gross margin percentage). Unless specifically stated as a percent of cost, markup is assumed to be a percentage of the selling price.

Mark-up % on cost = (Selling price – Acquisition cost) ÷ Acquisition cost

Mark-up on retail = (Selling price – Acquisition cost) ÷ Selling price

Example:

Assume that a pharmacy purchases merchandise for $80 and sells it for $100. What is the mark-up? What is the % mark-up on cost? What is the % mark-up on retail?

Mark-up = $100 -$80 or $20

Mark-up % on cost = [($100 -$80) ÷ $80] x 100
= ($20 ÷ $80) x 100
= 25%

Mark-up % on retail = [($100 -$80) ÷ $100] x 100
= ($20 ÷ $100) x 100
= 20%

Inventory turnover rate (ITOR). The inventory turnover rate is a measure of how fast inventory is being sold. ITOR can be calculated as the number of times per year that the average amount of inventory on hand at any given time is sold over the course of a year. It can also be calculated as the average number of days that it takes to sell the average amount of merchandise carried by the pharmacy.

The ITOR for a community pharmacy is calculated as the pharmacy's cost for the merchandise that it sold during the year (i.e., COGS) divided by the average amount of inventory that it had in stock during the year.

ITOR = COGS ÷ Average inventory*

*Average inventory is often estimated as the pharmacy's beginning inventory plus its ending inventory divided by 2.

To determine the number of days for inventory to turn over, divide 365 by the ITOR. Because they don't have sales *per se*, hospitals often find it useful to calculate ITOR as the amount of annual inventory purchases divided by average inventory.

Hospital ITOR = Purchases ÷ Average inventory

In 2005 the average retail pharmacy has an ITOR of just over 10 times (i.e., inventory is turned over approximately every 36.5 days). Hospitals usually have a much higher ITOR than community pharmacies because they are able to stock a smaller variety of drugs within each therapeutic class.

DOSAGE UNITS AND DAYS SUPPLY

As a pharmacy technician, you will frequently calculate how much medication you should dispense or the number of days that a prescription will last. Following are some examples:

1. For practice, calculate the amount of Amoxicillin you would need to fill this prescription:

    Amoxicillin 250 mg/5 mL
    Sig: ʒ i tid x 10 days
    By reading the prescription, you know that:
    Dosage = ʒ i = 5 mL
    Frequency = tid = 3 times a day
    Duration = 10 days
    So the order "ʒ i tid x 10 days" calls for 5 mL three times a day, for 10 days.

    Therefore, you would need 150 mL of Amoxicillin (5 mL x 3 times a day x 10 days).

2. Assume that the above prescription calls for 5 ounces of medication. How many grams of amoxicillin would the prescription contain?

mL/dose =   5 mL (see above)
Total quantity (in mL) =   5 fluid ounces x 30 mL/oz = 150 mL
Doses per bottle =   150 mL/bottle ÷ 5mL/dose = 30
doses mg/bottle =   250 mg/dose x 30 doses = 7,500 mg
grams/bottle =   7,500 mg ÷ 1,000 = 7.5 grams

Therefore, 7.5 grams of amoxicillin are contained in the prescription.

3. If the pharmacy purchases a one-pound jar of ointment, how many 60-gram prescriptions can be made from this amount?

Convert pounds to grams: One pound = 480 g

Divide total grams by grams per prescription: 480 g ÷ 60 g/Rx = 8 Rxs
Or
Convert pounds to ounces: One pound = 16 oz.
Convert grams to ounces: 30 g = one ounce
Determine number of ounces per prescription: 60 g/Rx ÷ 30g/oz = 2 oz/Rx
Divide total ounces by ounces per prescription: 16 oz ÷ 2 oz/Rx = 8 Rxs

Therefore, the one-pound jar could be used to make eight two-ounce prescriptions.

3. ℞   Proventil® Syrup
          Sig: ii tsp qid
          Disp 8 oz
          a) What is the daily dose?
          b) How long will the prescription last?
          Dosage = 2 tsp. = 10 mL
          Frequency = qid = 4 times a day
          Daily dose = 10 mL/dose x 4 doses/day = 40 mL/day
          Number of mL dispensed = 8 oz x 30 mL/oz. = 240 mL
          Day's supply = mL dispensed ÷ daily dose
          = 240mL ÷ 40 mL
          = 6 days.

4. ℞   Depakene® 250 mg tabs
          Sig: 0.5 gm qid for one month
          What quantity should be
          dispensed? Dosage = 500 mg
          Number of tablets per dose = 500 mg/dose ÷ 250 mg/tablet = 2 tablets
          Frequency = qid = 4 times a day
          Duration =30 days

Therefore, 2 tablets per dose x 4 doses/day x 30 days = 240 tablets

SELF-ASSESSMENT QUESTIONS CHAPTER V

1. A prescription calls for 200 mg of a drug, which is available as a concentration of 250 mg/5 mL. How many mL of this solution do you need?

2. A prescription reads Cefzil 500 mg q6h for 10 days. You have available to you 250 mg/5 mL of Cefzil. What quantity is needed to fill the entire prescription?

3. The dose for a medication reads to administer 25 mg/kg as a one-time dose. We have a patient who weighs 35 lbs. How much medication would we give this patient?

4. You have a 50 mg/mL concentration of a drug. Your prescription requires 400 mg of the drug, how many mL will you need?

5. Drug X is available in a concentration of 2 mg/15 mL, and your prescription calls for 10 mg of the drug. How many mL will you need?

6. A prescription is ordered which requires 10 mEq KCl and 15 mEq of K Acetate in 1000 mL D5W to be administered over 8 hours. What is the rate in mL/min?

7. Drug X is available in a concentration of 50 mcg/mL and the prescription calls for 0.24 mg of the drug. How many mL are required.

8. Convert 1:20 (w/v) to a %

9. Convert the following:
   a. 50 kg   =   _mg
   b. 100 mL   =   _L

10. Convert the following fractions to percents:
    a. 1/8   =   _____%
    b. 25/1000   =   _____%

11. Convert the following percents to decimals
    a. 34%   =   ___
    b. 4.5%   =   ___

12. You have 70% dextrose solution how many grams of dextrose are in 75 mL?

13. If 6 tablets cost $13.00, then how much will it cost for 15 tablets?

14. The cost of human growth hormone is $40/mg. What is the yearly cost of treating a 30 kg child at a dose of 0.04 mg/kg/day?

15. ℞ Prednisone 5 mg
    Sig: 2 tabs qid x 2 days
          2 tabs tid x 2 days
          2 tabs bid x 2 days
          1 tab tid x 2 days
          1 tab bid x 2 days Then stop. Qty qs

    What quantity should be dispensed?

16. ℞ Bactrim® Susp
Sig: 5 mL qid for 10 days

   a. What quantity should be dispensed?
   b. In what size bottle should this prescription be dispensed?

17. ℞ Cyclobenzaprine 10 mg tabs
Sig: 20 mg qid x 5 days

What quantity should be dispensed?

18. A formula for 1 L of a liquid pharmaceutical calls for 0.25 grams of methyl-paraben, a preservative. Approximately how many mg of this preservative are needed to make 1 pint of the liquid?
   a. 0.118 mg.
   b. 118 mg.
   c. 11.8 mg.
   d. 75 mg.

19. ℞ Proventil® Syrup
Sig: ii tsp quid
Disp. 8 oz

How many days supply will be dispensed?
a. 2 days.
b. 84 days.
c. 6 days.
d. 12 days.

20. 9.2 g equals:
   a. 920 mg.
   b. 9,200 mg.
   c. 92,000 mcg.
   d. 920,000 mcg.

21. One cubic centimeter (cc) is equal to:
   a. 0.001 liter.
   b. 0.01 liter.
   c. 0.1 liter.
   d. 1000 milliliters.

22. One pint equals:
   a. 12 fluid oz.
   b. 8 fluid oz.
   c. 473 mL.
   d. 240 mL.

23. Assume that drug cost (COGS) = $16 and selling price is $20.

    a. What is the markup in dollars?

    b. What is the percent markup on retail?

    c. What is the percent markup on cost?

24. Given:

Pharmacy Sales	$900,000
Cost of Goods Sold	$750,000
Beginning Inventory	$100,000
Ending Inventory	$50,000

    a. What is the Gross Margin as a percentage of sales?

    b. What is the Inventory Turnover Rate?

Answers:
1) 4 mL
2) 400 mL
3) 400 mg
4) 8 mL
5) 75 mL
6) 2 mL/min
7) 4.8 mL
8) 5 %
9a) 50,000,000 mg
9b) 0.1 L
10a) 12.5%
10b) 2.5 %
11a) 0.34
11b) 0.045
12) 52.5 g
13) $ 32.50
14) $ 17,520
15) 2 tabs/dose x 4 doses/day x 2 days = 8 tabs/day x 2 days = 16 tabs
    2 tabs/dose x 3 doses/day x 2 days = 6 tabs/day x 2 days = 12 tabs
    2 tabs/dose x 2 doses/day x 2 days = 4 tabs/day x 2 days = 8 tabs
    1 tab /dose x 3 doses/day x 2 days = 3 tabs/day x 2 days = 6 tabs
    1 tab /dose x 2 doses/day x 2 days = 2 tabs/day x 2 days = 4 tabs
        Dispense: 46 tabs total
16a) 5 mL/dose x 4 doses/day x 10 days = 200 mL
16b) 200 mL ÷ 30 mL/oz = 6.7 oz. Therefore, use an eight ounce bottle (the smallest size that will hold 200 mL)
17) 2 tabs/dose x 4 doses/day x 5 days = 40 tablets
18) b
19) c
20) b
21) a
22) c
23a) $4
23b) 20%
23c) 25%
24a) 16.7%
24b) 10

PHARMACY TECHNICIAN COMPETENCY ASSESSMENT
CHAPTER V

| Description of Ability or Skill | Initials | | Training Completed | |
	Tech	R.Ph.	Date	Remarks
The technician trainee has demonstrated knowledge of the terms and units of measurement in each of the systems of measurement and can convert from one system to another.				
The technician trainee is able to use Roman numerals.				
The technician trainee is able to correctly calculate ratios and proportions, dilutions of stock solutions and percentage preparations.				
The technician trainee is able to correctly calculate percentage preparations.				
The technician trainee is able to correctly calculate IV flow rates and infusion times.				
The technician trainee is able to correctly calculate prescription quantities and days supply.				
The technician trainee is able to convert from one system of temperature measurement to another.				
The technician trainee is able to perform basic business calculations.				

Chapter VI
Patient Interaction

EDUCATIONAL OBJECTIVES

After studying the material in this chapter, the technician trainee should be able to:

- Describe the importance of maintaining a caring attitude with patients
- Understand communication techniques to use with patients
- Describe the pharmacy department's policy on professional appearance
- Use effective telephone communication strategies
- Communicate patients' telephone requests to pharmacists
- Recognize the prescription-related telephone calls a technician cannot handle

---

COMMUNICATING WITH PATIENTS IN THE PHARMACY

Sometimes you work behind the scenes in the pharmacy department; sometimes you work face-to-face with patients. Both kinds of tasks are important because they improve patient service. Your behind-the-scenes work relieves pharmacists of some of their tasks, giving them more time to counsel patients about medications and perform other professional services. Your face-to-face work with patients, gathering information or completing their prescription transaction, serves the patient more directly. When you work directly with patients, you represent the pharmacy, and its reputation rests with you. When patients talk to you, they should know that you are interested, and that they are in capable, courteous hands.

So, whom do you serve: pharmacists or patients? The answer is both. Balancing your time is one of the most important skills required of pharmacy technicians. You cannot sacrifice serving patients to complete your behind-the-counter work. Yet, you cannot ignore your duties behind the counter because doing so obstructs the pharmacy's work flow. This chapter describes patient service at the counter and on the telephone and explains why these services are important and how you can best serve the people who enter your pharmacy.

The Importance of Personal Service

Question: How important is the personal service you offer?

Answer: Extremely. Many customers choose a particular pharmacy because of its service. Many of your pharmacy's patients may find that your pharmacy's staff makes patients feel confident that they receive excellent care. To many patients, picking up their medication is an extension of visiting their doctor; it is an important part of their health care, and they want to interact with pleasant people whom they trust.

People expect personal, caring attention in a pharmacy. The prescription they are getting is their medication, prescribed specifically for them. This is not a purchase in the same sense as buying a bottle of mouthwash—this purchase has their name on it. And if the prescription is new, patients may be concerned with how to take it, its possible side effects, and its interactions with other medications they may already take.

While only pharmacists may answer patients' questions and counsel them on how to take medications, you are part of the purchase process. You greet the patient, you fill out the information needed on the prescription, and you set the tone for the transaction. Pharmacists generally counsel patients after prescriptions are filled. However, you may be expected to complete the transaction by ringing up the sale. In that sense, you are the first and last impression patients carry with them. Because of this, not even the most helpful pharmacist can undo the damage that could result from a technician's negligence, impatience, or indifference.

By hiring you, pharmacists are trusting you with their business. You must make people feel welcome, well-served, and appreciated. You must also respect patients' privacy, time, questions, and feelings.

Question: What happens if you do not meet patients' expectations?

Answer: These patients will take their business elsewhere. But they will not do it silently.

Dissatisfied patients are much more likely to tell others about their experience than are satisfied patients. While good word-of-mouth advertising helps the pharmacy's reputation in the community, complaints travel further. Think about the bad experiences you have had in stores and how memorable they are. Research indicates that the number one reason people quit patronizing a particular pharmacy is because of a bad experience with a staff member.

Relationship with Patients

You can provide good patient service by building a rapport with each patient and by understanding the patient-pharmacy staff relationship.

Patients are the most important people in your day. Patients depend on the pharmacy

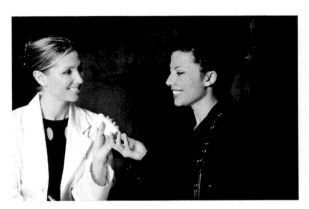

department for service. More importantly, the staff must remember that the pharmacy department depends on patients for its existence. Patients choose your pharmacy and honor it with their prescription business. "Honor" is not too strong a word. The plain fact is this: in a competitive marketplace, patients do the pharmacy a favor by coming in. Therefore, in serving patients, you must offer courteous and attentive service. Whether the patient is the first person you serve in the day or the last, young or old, courteous or rude, your challenge is to satisfy each patient's needs.

Patients are never an interruption. While you may be busy behind the counter with several demanding tasks, you cannot think of patients waiting at the counter as interruptions. Filing, data entry, stocking, and returning medication to the shelves are important parts of your routine. Yet, those jobs must be set aside to take care of patients. Each patient is a person who, most likely, is ill or in pain and who needs your help.

Your goal is to meet patients' needs and wants with a caring attitude. You have heard the slogan, "The customer is always right." That spirit should guide your work. What that slogan really says is that your job is to meet patients' needs and wants. Sometimes, doing so requires creativity, especially during situations such as the following:

- When patients do not understand that their prescriber must be called before you can fill a prescription
- When patients feel they are not being taken care of quickly enough
- When patients get confused about insurance coverage information

These are times when a caring attitude, your tone of voice, your eye contact, and the words you choose can communicate to the patient, "We will take care of you here. You are going to be all right."

Delivering superior patient service is not always easy. You may be under pressure to serve five or six people who happen to enter the pharmacy at once, and some people may be slow to understand or have difficulty hearing. Moreover, all of the quirks and flaws of human nature can be magnified when treating patients who are not feeling well. All of these challenges are part of serving people as a member of a health profession.

Developing a Caring Attitude

Question: What sets your pharmacy department apart from the others in your area?
Answer: The caring attitude with which you and your co-workers serve patients.

Greet patients warmly. When patients enter the prescription area, always welcome them with a smile and a few words of greeting, "Hello. How may I help you?" If you know a patient's name, use it. People like being recognized, yet they have grown accustomed to a marketplace that has reduced doing business to account numbers and fast, anonymous, and frequently rude service. That is why remembering and using a name adds a rare and impressive personal touch.

> "Hello, Mrs. Morgan. How are you today?" or
> "Hello, Mr. Davis. How may I help you today?"

Because many patients come regularly to the pharmacy department, you will quickly learn to attach names to faces. However, never take the liberty of addressing a patient by his or her first name unless invited to do so. All business and professional relationships should maintain a degree of formality.

Establish rapport with patients. After you greet patients, continue to emphasize the personal dimension of your service by looking directly into their eyes while you talk. Doing so shows you are giving them your undivided attention.

Listen to the tone of your voice. Is it warm and friendly, or is it stressed and abrupt, perhaps reflecting the pressures of a busy day? How are you holding your body? Is your stance challenging or impatient, as if saying "Oh, no. Here comes another problem. What will this patient want?" Are you scowling, or is your body relaxed and welcoming? Professionals do not let their stress show. After all, patients are not responsible for whatever is troubling you. If you look hurried or stressed, patients may wonder if you are going to take your exasperation out on them or if your mood will interfere with your job.

By building a rapport with patients, you give them a feeling of importance. Your actions say, "We appreciate your coming to our pharmacy department. We care about you."

Communicate with patients even if you are busy. If you cannot take care of patients immediately, acknowledge them in a warm, friendly tone and say, "I will be with you in a moment," or "I am just finishing up here. It will only be a minute." After you finish your phone conversation or take care of other patients, look the waiting patient directly in the eye, and say something like, "Now, how may I help you today?" Waiting patients should feel that now it is their turn to be served, and you will not cheat them to hurry on to other patients.

Note: Never keep patients waiting while you finish a routine project, like filing papers or putting away an incoming order of medication. Patients always come first. Their business pays your salary. Serving them is critical to the pharmacy department's security in the marketplace.

DISPENSING ERRORS

What Constitutes an Error?

A medication error is any preventable event that may cause or lead to inappropriate medication use or patient harm while the medication is in the control of the health care professional, patient, or consumer. It is important to minimize dispensing errors. Well-trained pharmacy technicians can help pharmacies avoid problems by being careful and alert. If you see something that doesn't look right, you have a responsibility to bring this to the attention of the pharmacist. You and the pharmacist also have the responsibility for detecting system problems that allow errors to happen and taking action to improve these systems so that the same type of error is less likely to occur in the future.

To be dispensed correctly, the prescription must be for the right drug, dispensed to the right patient at the right time with the right instructions. Many things can go wrong; therefore, there are many types of errors. A dispensing error can be the wrong drug, wrong strength, wrong dosage form or the wrong directions. In a hospital setting, doses that are given to patients behind schedule are counted as errors.

Be especially careful of look-alike and sound-alike drug names (see the sections titled "Distinguishing Among Easily Confused Products" and "Examples of Look-Alike or Sound-Alike Medication Names" in Chapter II). Also be careful of abbreviations that can easily be misinterpreted (see the section titled "Potential Misinterpretations of Abbreviations in Chapter IV). An error can also involve the dispensing to the wrong person or dispensing at the wrong time. Although the most obvious type of dispensing error is a prescription misfill, there are many other potential problems such as:

- Losing a phone-in order
- Failing to provide expanded service such as monitoring and counseling
- Being overly aggressive on a controlled substance prescription to the point of offensiveness
- Disclosing private medical information
- Dispensing a generic product from a DAW-signed prescription
- Stepping out of bounds by doing jobs that should be handled by pharmacist only
- Failing to fulfill deadlines as promised

The leading causes of errors are failure to be attentive and failure to follow approved procedures and protocols. What causes technicians to be inattentive or fail to follow approved procedures? Two of the more common factors that lead to inattentiveness or failure to follow procedures are distractions and improper training. The pharmacy department should minimize distractions by maintaining a work area that is free of clutter and free from unnecessary noise and interruptions. Training should be on-going and should focus on improving those areas that are identified as weaknesses. As an example, this on-going training could include periodic staff meetings to discuss potential problems and ways that they can be avoided. All pharmacy technicians should be well-trained and should be able to recognize errors and know how to prevent them.

Nevertheless, it is important to recognize that even in the most well-designed systems with the best-trained personnel, errors can still happen. All personnel must be willing to face these mistakes and even near-mistakes and learn from them. A very important part of an error prevention program is recognizing the importance of reporting any errors or near errors so that they can be addressed and resolved as soon as possible. Documenting errors will help the pharmacy department identify systems problems that can be improved in order to minimize errors in the future. These issues are discussed in more detail below.

Reporting and Responsibilities Regarding Errors

It is important that you approach an error with the correct attitude to manage the error and fix the problem, not with an attitude of panic. It is vitally important to notify the pharmacist of the problem as soon as it is detected. It's a good idea to use a code phase when telling pharmacist about a medication error. For example, "I have an urgent matter to address with you." This way the pharmacist will know that his or her attention is needed right away without alarming all the patients and other staff who may be nearby. Also, when discussing the matter, do so in an office or other private space in the pharmacy that creates a comfortable confidential environment.

Pharmacy technicians are responsible for reporting all errors to their pharmacist supervisor. It's a good idea to also report near-errors. Rather than assessing blame for making errors, the pharmacist supervisor should encourage reporting and focus on the system problems rather than disciplining individuals. Technicians should NEVER attempt to hide an error or decide for themselves whether an error is serious or not. Failure to report errors should be considered to be a serious breach of professional standards and should not be tolerated under any circumstances.

Documenting Errors

Your pharmacy will probably have a policy and procedure for documenting errors. Most likely, it will be your pharmacy supervisor who will complete the incident report or do the proper documentation. The primary reason for documenting errors is to detect trends or problems that can be corrected in the future. For example, assume that a pharmacist detected a potential problem with a prescription and was waiting for a call back from a physician before dispensing the prescription. If another technician or pharmacist was unaware that there was an unresolved problem, it is possible that the prescription could be completed and dispensed anyway. By detecting this problem, the pharmacy staff could design a policy and procedure for handling prescriptions that were awaiting a physician call back. This could vary from moving the prescription order to a separate work area, attaching a note to the prescription order, or locking the computer so a label could not be printed without proper authorization. Be sure to ask your pharmacist supervisor about the proper procedure for documenting errors in your pharmacy.

Handling Problems

Adopting a positive attitude means that you do not offer excuses or lay blame on someone else when things go wrong. Sometimes prescriptions are not ready on time, prescriptions get misplaced, or patients are overcharged. Even more serious, however, is an error with the label, drug, strength or dosage form accidentally given to a patient. These are examples of "critical moments." These moments must be handled expertly and professionally so the pharmacist-patient relationship is not harmed.

> **Note:** Inform a pharmacist immediately of any misfills or other serious problems. Do not try to handle the situation yourself.

Prepare for critical moments because they happen unexpectedly. While you will learn how to handle lesser critical concerns, like those involving a prescription that is not ready on time or an overcharge, only a pharmacist should handle the more serious moments.

Since the pharmacy staff has little time to think about reacting to critical moments, following the pattern outlined below will help you cope with the situation.

- **Listen to the patient's entire story.** Just listening without interrupting the patient will help diffuse the situation. Usually that means listening until the patient stops speaking and the emotional outburst passes.

- **Echo the patient's points, showing that you care and identify with the problem.** Sometimes called "reflective listening," this technique feeds back to patients what has just been told to you.

- **Use a calm tone and relaxed body language.** Look patients in the eye and assure them of your genuine regret about the problem. Keep your body relaxed. This signals that you know how to take care of the situation.

  Research shows that words carry only about ten to 15 percent of spoken messages. The rest is delivered in the tone of voice (about 35 percent), and by the posture and gestures (about 50 percent) accompanying the words. Unless we master and orchestrate all three of these communication signals, we may send contradictory messages. Our facial expressions and body language may signal the opposite of what our words say.

- **Do not make excuses.** Do not try to defend how the mistake may have happened. Being busy is no excuse. New employees or a short-staffed pharmacy department are also not excuses. Having a head cold and not being able to think clearly is no excuse. Excuses send two messages:

  1. We may have done it, but it is not our fault; and
  2. We are sometimes out of control in this pharmacy department.

The first message is wrong—mistakes are the pharmacy department's fault. Typically, patients want apologies, not a defense of your pharmacy department. The second message is a dangerous one—it undermines patients' confidence in your pharmacy department's ability to do its job.

- **Do not argue.** This is not a battle of wits or a competition. Avoid rudeness and sarcasm at all costs. Listen until patients finish their story. Then try to offer constructive solutions.

- **Do not try to minimize the problem.** By implying that the problem really is not so bad, you will probably only infuriate the patient. You will trivialize the trouble. Patients want you to recognize and respect their problems.

- **If possible, assure the patient you will find the cause of the problem.** Promise that you will discover how it happened to prevent it from happening again. Tell the patient that you are sorry for the trouble.

- **Resolve the problem as positively as possible.** You can correct overcharges on a prescription right away and immediately prepare a prescription that was not filled before its scheduled pick-up time. If you are unable to resolve the problem, refer it to the pharmacist.

Handled correctly, critical moments can become opportunities to improve patient relations. Usually patients will accept your willingness to cooperate with them and to make amends if you take complaints seriously, express the pharmacy department's regret, and act immediately to resolve problems.

Note: Here is an example of a critical moment you might have to handle:

An obviously frustrated patient steps up to the counter and tells you that he has been trying to call the pharmacy department for the last 45 minutes to request a refill. The patient needs the prescription today and has to be at work within the hour. The patient is angry about the time wasted redialing and is looking for an argument.

After you have let the patient "vent" by telling his story without interruption, show that you understand by calmly echoing the patient's feelings. "I am sorry for the inconvenience. I know how frustrating a busy signal can be." Next, take immediate action to solve the problem. "I will give this to the pharmacist immediately. It will be the next prescription filled and should only take a few minutes." You have solved the patient's problem quickly and easily and he should feel well served.

One of the most important aspects of your job is serving people warmly and courteously. Patient satisfaction, more than low prices or flashy promotions, results in loyal return customers.

YOUR PERSONAL APPEARANCE

While warmth and courtesy are essential, your appearance has to blend in with a team of professionals. Moreover, because you are a member of a health care team, you must look and act professionally. What does that mean? You must dress appropriately. The pharmacy department's policy and procedure manual may cover this in more detail.

Clothing. You may wear a white pharmacy jacket, but the blouse or shirt beneath that jacket will still show. It should not be too casual or too wildly colorful. Trousers or skirts should also be appropriate to the workplace—blue jeans and shorts, for example, are usually inappropriate in a professional setting.

Clean, well-styled hair. Hairstyles should be neat and controlled.

Food. A business-like, professional appearance means that you do not eat food or snacks or drink beverages while patients can see you. Likewise, you should not chew gum, or eat candy.

COMMUNICATING ON THE TELEPHONE

All the patient service principles that apply to face-to-face service also apply to telephone service. Every time you answer the phone or place a call, you represent your pharmacy department to the patient on the other end of the line. Your attitude is clearly communicated in your voice.

Actually, you may have to work harder at telephone communications than at serving people at the counter. When people can see your face, your smile, and the attention in your eyes, you send many warm, visual signals. However, on the telephone, with all visual signals removed, your voice becomes more important; you must use it to deliver your message in a manner, tone, and speed that is friendly and inviting. To some patients, your voice is their pharmacy.

General Guidelines for Telephone Use

Many incoming calls will concern prescriptions. These calls may originate from prescribers' offices or from patients needing new or refill prescriptions. Whenever calls do not need the attention of a pharmacist, you will probably be asked to handle them. Here are some general guidelines for answering the phone:

Answer the phone promptly, by the third ring. Doing so projects an image of efficiency.

- Immediately identify your store, your department, your name, your position and offer a service. For example: "Brown Drugs, Prescription Department. This is Janet, the pharmacy technician. May I help you?"

- Give the caller a chance to speak. Be alert and give your full attention to the person who is calling. Do not interrupt, and do not become distracted by what is going on around you in the store.

- Speak clearly and distinctly.

- Show interest in the tone of your voice. Be pleasant, but sound natural.

- Speak at a moderate speed, so callers can follow the conversation.

If you can handle the call yourself, give the caller the information quickly, politely, and professionally. If you must leave the telephone to get information, be courteous and say, "Let me check on that for you. Can you hold please?" Then use the hold button if your phone has one. If not, gently set the receiver down and get the information. When you return, begin by saying, "Thank you for waiting. I have that information for you now." When you finish your conversation, thank the patient for calling, and remember to replace the receiver gently when you hang up.

If the caller needs another department, explain that another staff member can help the caller. Tell the caller you will transfer the call, saying something like, "The manager can answer your question. I will transfer you." Put the call on hold and notify the manager that a call is waiting. Stay alert to the flashing hold button and the manager's whereabouts to be sure that the manager does not get distracted and forget the caller.

If the call is for a pharmacist, tell the caller, "Just one moment, please. The pharmacist will help you with that." Put the caller on hold, and tell the pharmacist that the caller is waiting. Again, keep an eye on the blinking hold button to be sure the pharmacist does not forget about the caller.

Prescription-Related Calls You Can Handle

Many of the incoming calls to the prescription department will not need to be given to a pharmacist; you can take care of these callers' needs.

Patients who call ahead to confirm their prescriptions are ready. Always check. Simply because prescriptions were dropped off in the morning does not necessarily mean they will be ready in the afternoon. Put the callers on hold and locate their prescriptions in your pharmacy department's pick-up area. Then return to the telephone to tell them whether their prescriptions are ready.

Patients who want to transfer existing prescriptions to the pharmacy. These patients may be new to your area, or they may simply have decided to change pharmacies. Whatever the reason, the procedure is the same. Even though the prescription exists at another pharmacy, it must be treated like a new prescription (which it is for your pharmacy department).

In transferring prescriptions from one pharmacy to another, getting both the prescriber and pharmacy department information is important. Your pharmacist must call the pharmacy department where the prescription was last filled to get information about the medication.

Patients who call in refills. Record the same refill information as you would if the patient came to the pharmacy department. It is a good idea to ask for telephone numbers where patients can be reached so a pharmacist can contact patients when necessary. Also, ask patients when they will pick up the prescription. This gives pharmacists a working deadline and saves patients a wasted trip. If prescriptions cannot be ready by this time, call them to arrange a new pick-up time.

Patients who have no more refills and ask you to call their doctor. Pharmacists should call as soon as possible, giving the prescriber plenty of time to return the call, if necessary. By giving prescribers enough lead time, the pharmacy department will be better able to meet patients' requested pick-up times. In some states technicians may be able to contact prescribers for refill authorization. Check with a pharmacist.

Incoming Calls You Cannot Handle

There are several kinds of calls that should be handled by a pharmacist. It is important to know the limits of your duties as a pharmacy technician. There are some types of telephone calls that you are not allowed to handle and they must be referred to a pharmacist:

- ***Prescribers' calls.*** Whenever prescribers' offices call about anything that you are not allowed to handle, be courteous and tell the callers that you will transfer them to a pharmacist. Say something like, "Just a moment please. I will get the pharmacist for you."

- ***Informational/emergency calls.*** Callers who have questions about side effects, overdoses, and poisons must be transferred to a pharmacist immediately.

- ***Calls from other pharmacies.*** On occasion, pharmacists from another pharmacy will call to transfer a prescription. Pharmacy technicians are not allowed to handle these calls in most states.

- ***Calls about prescription errors.*** Despite the pharmacy department's hard work, mistakes may happen. You may receive a call from a patient who says a mistake has been made in filling a prescription. The error could be a harmless embarrassment or a life-threatening situation requiring hospitalization, and may involve possible lawsuits. These calls should only be handled by a pharmacist. Simply stating, "I will give you to the pharmacist," is sufficient. Put the caller on hold, and explain the nature of the call to the pharmacist. You can help pharmacists handle these calls by preparing the information that they will need to talk with the patient. Pull up the patient's profile or the prescription price in question so that the pharmacist has the needed background for the telephone conversation.

The statement at the beginning of this chapter—that patients are the most important people in your day—is not an exaggeration. They are the most important people in the day for everyone working in the pharmacy. And providing them with the careful attention and quality service they need and deserve is made possible in large part by all the work that you do as a technician. You are as important to good patient care as anyone on the pharmacy staff. After all, you have as much, possibly more, face-to-face contact with patients as anyone. You also work to make sure that the supplies needed to process prescriptions are available so that patients' needs are met immediately. Everything you do ensures that patients get the best care possible.

SELF-ASSESSMENT QUESTIONS CHAPTER VI

1. When you are busy working with one patient and notice that several others are now waiting at the prescription counter, you should:
   a. Finish working with the patient as fast as possible and then work as quickly as possible with each of the other patients.
   b. Ask the pharmacist to wait on the patients.
   c. Suggest that the patients come back later when it is not quite so busy.
   d. Acknowledge the patients' presence and let them know that you will wait on each of them soon.

2. Research shows that when people speak, most of the message is carried by:
   a. Words.
   b. Tone of voice.
   c. Posture and gestures accompanying the words.
   d. Physical appearance.

3. Which of the following excuses are acceptable when a mistake has been made?
   a. Being busy.
   b. New employees.
   c. Short-staffed pharmacy department.
   d. None of the above.

4. Which of the following telephone calls should NOT be handled by a pharmacy technician?
   a. Patients calling to transfer existing prescriptions to the pharmacy.
   b. Patients calling in refills.
   c. Patients who have no more refills and ask you to call their doctor.
   d. Prescribers' calls.

5. According to the *Training Program,* which of the following is true regarding use of the telephone?
   a. Answer the telephone before it rings a second time.
   b. Finish the job you are doing before answering the telephone.
   c. When answering the telephone, identify your store, your department, your name, and your position.
   d. Minimize the time it takes to talk on the telephone by reminding the caller that you are very busy.

Answers:
1) d
2) c
3) d
4) d
5) c

PHARMACY TECHNICIAN COMPETENCY ASSESSMENT

CHAPTER VI

Description of Ability or Skill	Initials		Training Completed	
	Tech	R.Ph.	Date	Remarks
The technician trainee understands and can explain the importance of establishing and maintaining a caring attitude with patients.				
The technician trainee uses proper communication techniques with patients.				
The technician trainee understands the importance of maintaining a professional personal appearance and can describe the pharmacy department's policy on this issue.				
The technician trainee uses effective telephone communication skills.				
The technician trainee effectively communicates patients' telephone requests to pharmacists.				
The technician trainee knows and can describe the prescription-related telephone calls a technician cannot handle.				

Chapter VII
An Overview of Federal Privacy Requirements

By: Deborah Faucette, R.Ph.

EDUCATIONAL OBJECTIVES

After reviewing materials contained in this chapter, the technician trainee should be able to:

- Understand the main concepts of the federal privacy rules that impact the technician role
- Describe certain procedures that must be followed during the dispensing process to comply with the privacy regulations
- Communicate with patients and healthcare professionals in compliance with the privacy rules
- Effectively maintain privacy when communicating with those other than the patient
- Understand the basic patient rights as described in the privacy regulations which may affect the technician's role.

Important Note

This chapter is intended to provide an overview of the federal privacy rules, but it is not designed to satisfy the training requirement of the regulation. Your employer is responsible for training you on the specific privacy processes and procedures as developed by your particular company. In addition, this overview applies to the federal regulation only. Your particular state may have more stringent requirements in the area of patient privacy. Be sure to check for state specific requirements with your pharmacy manager or supervisor.

OVERVIEW

The Health Insurance Portability and Accountability Act of 1996 (HIPAA) is a very broad statute that covers a variety of healthcare issues. One portion of this law deals with the protection of the privacy of healthcare information, the Privacy Rule. Although these privacy regulations under HIPAA are quite complex, we will only address some of the components that may impact pharmacy technicians.

What is the Purpose of the Privacy Rules?

With the advancement of technology and the use of electronic records, the need arose to set some federal standards to protect personal healthcare information. Basically, the privacy rules outline how patients' protected health information can be used. Any healthcare provider that transmits electronic claims that contain protected health information is considered a **covered entity** and must comply with this regulation.

What is Protected Health Information (PHI)?

Protected health information (PHI) is any information that is collected at the pharmacy that can be used to identify a patient. Billing records, prescription records and patient profiles are all examples. In the pharmacy, PHI includes a patient's name, address, prescription number, telephone number, date of birth, and name of employer. It is this information that the privacy rules serve to protect.

IMPACT ON OPERATIONAL PROCEDURES IN THE PHARMACY

As a pharmacy technician, you are required to make reasonable efforts to comply with the privacy rules and safeguard Protected Health Information (PHI).

Let's take a few minutes just to review some areas in the dispensing process that will be affected by these new regulations:

Prescription Intake Area

You will need to remove protected health information whenever possible. Do not leave patient information lying around for others to see. For example, each empty vial or new prescription you collect from patients should be placed behind the counter out of the public eye as soon as it is received.

In addition, any questions you ask the patient to obtain information must be done as discreetly as possible. Speak in lower tones and away from other customers to protect the patient's information.

Prescription Outtake Area

Most pharmacies store completed prescriptions that are awaiting customer pick up in the "will call" section. In order to comply with protecting a patient's information, these bags with completed receipts should not be in plain view to the customer who steps up to the pharmacy counter.

In addition, you should keep the cash register area clear of any completed prescription vials other than those for the current patient. Even if the next person will be "right back," you will need to keep their PHI out of public view.

Notice of Privacy Practices

The Privacy Rule within HIPAA requires your pharmacy to provide each patient with a **Notice of Privacy Practices** the first time the pharmacy provides them a service.

The Notice of Privacy Practices is a multi-page document that is specific to your company and outlines for the patient all the ways their Protected Health Information (PHI) is used by the pharmacy. In addition, Patient Rights and the pharmacy's legal duties are outlined in the document. (A sample of a notice is posted at the end of this chapter.)

Therefore, the first time a patient receives medications or services from your pharmacy you must provide them a copy of your pharmacy's Notice. This only needs to be done once, but you can give it to the patient when they drop off the prescription to be filled or when the completed prescription is picked up. The Notice can also be placed in prescription bag of a completed prescription in the "will call" section.

The Privacy Rule also requires that your pharmacy have your Notice on hand to be given to anyone who asks for a copy. In addition, a copy of the pharmacy's Notice of Privacy Practices must be prominently posted in the pharmacy.

Acknowledgement Signatures

According to the privacy regulation, you must make a good faith effort to collect a patient's signature that acknowledges that they have received a copy of the Notice of Privacy Practices.

There are a variety of methods to collect this acknowledgement signature. For example, signatures can be recorded in the same logbook a customer already signs so long as the acknowledgement signature is on its own separate signature line.

Some pharmacies will also collect this acknowledgement signature through newer technology called electronic signature capture. This method usually involves an interface with the dispensing software so that the patient's profile is somehow flagged at the time that the acknowledgement signature is captured.

If someone other than the patient picks up the prescription, you may need to send an acknowledgement form home with the prescription. The patient can either mail back the signed form or drop it off at the pharmacy on the next visit. If a patient refuses to sign, you should still document the good-faith effort you made to obtain the acknowledgement signature.

Part of the privacy training you will receive from your employer will include specifically how you will handle the distribution of Notices and the collection of acknowledgement signatures. Ask your pharmacy manager or supervisor if you need any clarification.

Although you'll need to make some adjustments to perform these operational duties to comply with the Privacy Rules, they are not meant to prevent the pharmacy from filling a patient's prescription or providing other services. In other words, if a patient refuses to sign an acknowledgement, the pharmacy can still fill the prescription and consult with a patient.

Destruction of PHI

As a covered entity, your pharmacy is responsible for protecting your patients' health information. This includes information that leaves the pharmacy in the form of trash.

Any written patient information must be properly destroyed. Some pharmacies utilize shredders, whereas others keep pharmacy trash separately. Special precautions will need to be taken in order to comply with the Privacy Rule.

In addition to the "paper" trash, you'll need to take into account that old patient vials contain PHI and must be properly destroyed. Your pharmacy will provide you with information in proper destruction procedures that may include:

- Placing used vials in specially designated containers to be incinerated, or
- "Blacking out" PHI on the label with a permanent black marker (a bit labor intensive), or
- Giving the old vial back to the patient

IMPACT ON COMMUNICATIONS IN THE PHARMACY

Probably the biggest impact the Privacy Rule will have on your job performance is in the area of communication; in particular, verbal communications associated with good customer service.

Communications Associated With Good Customer Service

It will be critical for you to remember a rule while performing your job functions throughout the day: "keep it simple."

For example, in the past, you may have addressed a patient in this manner: "Mrs. Jones, I am sorry but your Imitrex® is not covered by your plan. Our pharmacist will have to call your physician for another drug for your migraines."

While this may sound polite and was intended to be helpful, too much protected health information is discussed. In addition, you do not want any private information overheard by another patient or customer. In order to provide that same level of service to your patients and yet comply with the Privacy Rules you'll want to address the situation with slight modifications by "keeping it simple."

"Mrs. Jones, our pharmacist will call your physician to ask for a prescription that is covered on your plan."

Of course, this dialogue is best conducted face to face away from other patients. You must make every effort to ensure that your conversations with patients are not overheard by others. Keep your voice low, and, if necessary, escort the patient away from other customers to enhance privacy.

Another procedure associated with good customer service is in properly notifying a patient that their prescription is ready. If your pharmacy utilizes some type of public address system to announce when a particular customer's prescription is ready, you'll want to double-check that procedure. Your company may decide to modify how the system is used to comply with the Privacy Rules. For instance, some companies' procedures involve stating, "Order for Jones is ready," refraining from using first names, physician names or drug names.

Communications with Coworkers

During the dispensing process, there are several occasions that may require discussion. For instance, if a clinical warning message appears alerting the pharmacist of a potential interaction, you'll need to bring it to the pharmacist's attention to render a decision.

You should "keep it simple" by limiting your verbal conversations to the minimum information possible. Rather than tell the pharmacist that "Mrs. Jones' new antibiotic may interfere with her Prozac®," you will need to keep the message to a simple notification to the pharmacist that he/she is needed to resolve a clinical issue.

As a general rule, you may want to refrain from using patient names in your discussions with coworkers whenever possible. You'll want to be cognizant of other customers in the store that may be in close proximity to your pharmacy. Although there may not be a patient right at the pharmacy counter, voices and conversations can carry and be overheard by other customers nearby.

Telephone Communications

You may be involved with obtaining or providing information with another healthcare provider, such as a physician's office. HIPAA rules were not intended to prevent the usual conversations regarding a patient's care between a pharmacist and physician. However, it will be necessary to conduct phone conversations so that patient privacy is preserved. Some pharmacies utilize portable phones, allowing pharmacists and technicians to walk to a more private area.

In addition, you will need to exercise caution before arbitrarily providing patient information to someone over the telephone.

Patient Counseling

The HIPAA Privacy Rules were not intended to impede the pharmacist's ability to counsel the patient. Under HIPAA, pharmacists will need to take every precaution to counsel a patient in a private area, using low tones so as not to be overheard by other patients nearby.

Communicating with a Third Party Present

In addition, certain precautions must be taken when a patient is in the presence of another acquaintance or when a person other than the patient picks up a prescription.

In the first instance, let's use the example of Mrs. Jones coming in to pick up her Imitrex® prescription, and she is accompanied by her son. Under the Privacy Rule, the pharmacist must take every precaution to restrict patient counseling to the person for whom it is intended. In this instance, a pharmacist can address this scenario and comply with the Privacy Rule by doing one of the following:

- Ask Mrs. Jones outright if it is okay to counsel her in front of her son
- Give the patient the opportunity to object to the conversation in front of her son
- Infer from her behavior that, based on the pharmacist's professional judgment, she does not object to receiving patient counseling in her son's presence

Other Special Circumstances

Consultations with Caregivers

Sometimes someone other than the patient arrives to pick up a prescription. Under the Privacy Rules, the pharmacist should use professional judgment in providing instruction and counseling information to that person. However, the information that the pharmacist provides needs to be limited to the minimum amount necessary that is relevant to that person's involvement in that patient's care. In other words, that person would not divulge the entire patient's profile, but limit the information provided to the caregiver to the prescription(s) being picked up at that time, and the patient's current condition, as in the best interests of the patient.

Minors

Each state has its own definition of a "minor." In some states, under the age of 18 may be the definition, where in others, it could be anyone under the age of 12. You will need to determine the criterion for a minor in your state, as it will affect your conduct with a customer.

You will not need to provide a Notice of Privacy Practices or obtain an acknowledgement signature with a minor, as this can be taken care of with the minor's parent or legal guardian. Check with your pharmacy manager or supervisor as to the proper procedure for engaging minors in your store.

Spouses

Although it has always been good professional practice to limit conversations to the patient present at the counter, HIPAA emphasizes this point to a greater extent.

In some instances, you might know that a spouse may be bedridden and cared for by the customer who comes to the counter to pick up the medication. But in most cases, you will not know and cannot assume. As a pharmacy technician, you may provide the customer the prescription they request to pick up, if it is for a spouse, but you should not discuss the prescription with the customer, deferring those questions to the pharmacist for the appropriate response.

As mentioned earlier, the pharmacist will use his or her professional judgment in the best interest of the patient, when it comes to counseling someone other than the patient. Before HIPAA was implemented, many pharmacies already had a procedure in place to protect a spouse's information. Many pharmacies will only supply copies of patient profiles when requested by the patients themselves, either in person or in writing.

INCIDENTAL DISCLOSURES

A **disclosure** occurs any time a patient's protected health information leaves your control and is provided elsewhere: to physician offices for treatment purposes, to third-party insurance companies for payment, or to an insurance clerk to re-bill a rejected claim. The above are all examples of disclosures that occur in the process of treatment, payment or operations of your organization.

However, sometimes protected health information is accidentally disclosed despite your good-faith attempt to keep it private. For example, a pharmacist might be overheard counseling a patient, even though the pharmacist spoke quietly to the patient. Such "incidental" disclosures do not violate the Privacy Rules as long as you have:

1. Followed your pharmacy's privacy policies and procedures;
2. Taken reasonable steps to prevent others from overhearing or seeing another patient's protected information; and
3. Disclosed only the "minimum necessary" amount of patient information (in situations where the "minimum necessary" rule applies).

PATIENT RIGHTS

The HIPAA Privacy Rule was designed to provide patients with greater control over their protected health information. The Notice of Privacy Practices, as written by the Privacy Rule, must outline a patient's rights and the process for acting upon those rights. For instance, the notice should provide patients the procedure for filing a complaint with the Department of Health and Human Services (the federal organization with jurisdiction over HIPAA) and a means to complain to the organization or pharmacy directly if they feel their privacy rights have been violated.

In addition, HIPAA provides patient rights in the following areas:

1. *The Right to Access Protected Health Information*

A patient has a right to receive a copy of his or her prescription profile. Be sure to check with the pharmacist before complying with a request; some pharmacies have a policy of requesting this in writing through a central location or "home office" rather than making store employees responsible. As mentioned earlier under disclosures, you should never give a copy of protected health information to anyone other than the patient, unless instructed to do so.

2. *The Right to Request Amendments of PHI*

A patient has the right to ask the pharmacy to change their profile information. For example, a patient may ask that their allergy to penicillin be added to their profile. In addition, a patient may ask that you delete a prescription from their records. A pharmacy may or may not make changes to the profile as requested by the patient. The pharmacy may deny the patient's request, using the procedures outlined in the Privacy Rule.

3. *The Right to Receive an Accounting of Disclosures*

Pharmacies are required to track certain non-routine disclosures of protected health information, such as disclosures of patient files to a board of pharmacy. Patients have the right to ask for an "accounting" of the pharmacy's non-routine disclosure of their protected health information.

4. *The Right to Request Additional Privacy*

A patient may ask that a pharmacy place additional restrictions on the release of the patient's protected health information. This occurs, for example, when a patient does not want you to bill their third-party insurance card and prefers to pay cash. For instance, Mrs. Jones may be taking medication in a sensitive situation (such as HIV) and my not want the information to go to the insurance company, fearing too many people will see the information. A pharmacy is under no obligation to agree to those restrictions, but must respond to the patient's request as outlined in the Privacy Rule.

120

5. *The Right to Request an Alternative Means of Communication*

A patient may ask that they be called at work, not at home, for refill reminders. A pharmacy will need to comply with all *reasonable* requests.

> **Note:** Your pharmacy will have specific policies and procedures in place for patients to exercise their rights. In some pharmacies, these requests may need to be in writing and may need to be sent directly to a central location. You'll need to check with your pharmacy to insure that you know what is expected of you.

EMPLOYER RESPONSIBILITIES

Under the HIPAA Privacy Rule, your employer's responsibilities are numerous. The following is just a short list of some of those responsibilities:

1. Developing written policies and procedures concerning privacy.
2. Appointing a **Privacy Officer** who is responsible to oversee the company's overall compliance with the HIPAA.
3. Training workforce members in privacy policies and procedures, as necessary to perform their job.
4. Responding to patient requests and complaints.
5. Maintaining reasonable safeguards to protected health information.
6. Settings up procedures for the complaint process, which must be outlined in the Notice of Privacy Practices.
7. Addressing employee concerns and enforcing sanctions against those who violate Privacy Rules.
8. Maintaining proper documentation as required by the Privacy Rule.

PENALTIES UNDER HIPAA

As mentioned in the previous section, your pharmacy is responsible for enforcing sanctions against individuals who violate the Privacy Rules. These sanctions may involve a verbal or written warning, suspension, or dismissal, depending upon the severity of the situation.

In addition, Health and Human Services (HHS) may impose civil penalties of $100 to $25,000 per violation of the Privacy Rule in any given year.

In addition to civil penalties, criminal violations can be imposed by the Department of Justice. Any person who obtains or discloses PHI in violation of the Privacy Rule can face a fine of $50,000 and up to one year in jail. This can increase to $100,000 and five years in prison if the PHI was obtained under false pretenses. In addition, a person who obtains PHI and intends to sell it for personal gain or malicious harm can face up to a $250,000 fine and ten years imprisonment.

EMPLOYEE RESPONSIBILITIES

As a member of the Pharmacy Team, you play a critical role in Privacy Rule compliance. You are the first person that the patient may see in the pharmacy and your courteous behavior will help to set the tone. You will also need to understand patients' rights under HIPAA, since you may be the first one a patient sees to inquire about those rights.

In addition, as an employee of your pharmacy, you have the responsibility of protecting your patients' information. Use the "minimum necessary" rule of "keeping it simple" so that you are not providing too much information.

The Privacy Rule also outlines that every employee should follow the company's privacy policies and procedures and should report any suspected violations of the Privacy Rule. Each pharmacy must implement a procedure for employees to report any suspected violations to the Privacy Officer.

While your role carries important responsibilities, these three things will help you follow the HIPAA rules:

1. Protect your patients' information using the "minimum necessary" rule.
2. Follow your pharmacy's privacy policies and procedures.
3. Report any suspected violations of the Privacy Rule to your Privacy Officer.

CONCLUSION

This chapter has provided you with the "bare bones" federal overview of the Privacy Rule within HIPAA. You will receive more specific information with regard to policies and procedures from your pharmacy. In addition, each state may have specific privacy requirements that are stricter than what is outlined here. You'll need to check with your pharmacy manager or supervisor to obtain the more specific company and/or state-required procedures.

EMPLOYEE CHECKLIST: PRIVACY PROCEDURES

Although your responsibilities may incorporate more procedures than what is outlined here, the following is a checklist of some of the procedures you should know to comply with the Privacy Rule:

1. How does your pharmacy provide the Notice of Privacy Practices to patients?

2. How does your pharmacy collect acknowledgement signatures?

3. How should you handle patient requests for access to PHI?

4. How should you handle patient requests for amendments to their PHI?

5. How should you handle patient requests for confidential communications?

6. How should you handle patient requests for accounting of disclosures?

7. How should you handle patient privacy complaints?

8. How should you dispose of PHI?

9. How should you report suspected violations of the privacy rule?

10. How do you get in contact with your Privacy Officer if you have questions or need clarification around procedures for privacy?

SAMPLE NOTICE OF PRIVACY FORM

NOTICE OF PRIVACY PRACTICES

This notice describes how medical information about you may be used and disclosed and how you can get access to this information. Please review it carefully.

The Pharmacy is required by law to maintain the privacy of your Protected Health Information ("PHI") and to provide individuals with you with a notice of our legal duties and privacy practices with respect to PHI. PHI is information about you, including basic demographic information, that may identify you and that relates to your past, present or future physical or mental health or condition and related health care services. This Notice of Privacy Practices ("Notice") describes how we may use and disclose PHI about you to carry out treatment, payment or health care operations and for other specified purposes that are permitted or required by law. The Notice also describes your rights with respect to PHI about you about you.

The Pharmacy is required to follow the terms of this Notice. We will not use or disclose PHI about you without your written authorization, except as described in this Notice. We reserve the right to change our practices and this Notice and to make the new Notice effective for all PHI we maintain. Upon request, we will provide any revised Notice to you.

Your Health Information Rights

You have the following rights with respect to PHI about you:

Obtain a paper copy of the Notice upon request. You may request a copy of the Notice at any time. Even if you have agreed to receive the Notice electronically, you are still entitled to a paper copy. To obtain a paper copy, contact _____.

Request a restriction on certain uses and disclosures of PHI. You have the right to request additional restrictions on our use or disclosure of PHI about you by sending a written request to _____. We are not required to agree to those restrictions.

Inspect and obtain a copy of PHI. You have the right to access and copy PHI about you contained in a designated record set for as long as the Pharmacy maintains the PHI. The designated record set usually will include prescription and billing records. To inspect or copy PHI about you, you must send a written request to _____. We may charge you a fee for the costs of copying, mailing and supplies that are necessary to fulfill your request. We may deny your request to inspect and copy in certain limited circumstances. If you are denied access to PHI about you, you may request that the denial be reviewed.

Request an amendment of PHI. If you feel that PHI we maintain about you is incomplete or incorrect, you may request that we amend it. You may request an amendment for as long as we maintain the PHI. To request an amendment, you must send a written request to. You must include a reason that supports your request. In certain cases, we may deny your request for amendment. If we deny your request for amendment, you have the right to file a statement of disagreement with the decision and we may give a rebuttal to your statement.

Receive an accounting of disclosures of PHI. You have the right to receive an accounting of the disclosures we have made of PHI about you after April 14, 2003 for most purposes other than treatment, payment, or health care operations. The accounting will exclude certain disclosures, such as disclosures we have made directly to you, disclosures you authorize, disclosures to friends or family members involved in your care, and disclosures for notification purposes. The right to receive an accounting is subject to certain other exceptions, restrictions, and limitations. To request an accounting, you must submit a request in writing to _____. Your request must specify the time period, but may not be longer than six years. The first accounting you request within a 12 month period will be provided free of charge, but you may be charged for the cost of providing additional accountings. We will notify you of the cost involved and you may choose to withdraw or modify your request at that time.

Request communications of PHI by a lternative means or at alternative locations. For instance, you may request that we contact you about medical matters only in writing or at a different residence or post office box. To request confidential communication of PHI about you, you must submit a request in writing to_____.
Your request must state how or where you would like to be contacted. We will accommodate all reasonable requests.

Examples of How We May Use and Disclose PHI
The following are descriptions and examples of ways we use and disclose PHI about you.

We will use PHI for treatment. Example: Information obtained by the pharmacist will be used to dispense prescription medications to you. We will document in your record information related to the medications dispensed to you and services provided to you.

We will use PHI for payment. Example: We will contact your insurer or pharmacy benefit manager to determine whether it will pay for your prescription and the amount of your copayment. We will bill you or a third-party payer for the cost of prescription medications dispensed to you. The information on or accompanying the bill may include information that identifies you, as well as the prescriptions you are taking.

We will use PHI for health care operations. Example: The Pharmacy may use information in your health record to monitor the performance of the pharmacists providing treatment to you. This information will be used in an effort to continually improve the quality and effectiveness of the health care and service we provide. We are likely to use or disclose PHI for the following purposes:

Business associates: There are some services provided by us through contracts with business associates. Examples include _____.
When these services are contracted for, we may disclose PHI about you to our business associate so that they can perform the job we have asked them to do and bill you or your third-party payer for services rendered. To protect PHI about you, we require the business associate to appropriately safeguard the PHI.

Communication with individuals involved in your care or payment for your care: Health professionals such as pharmacists, using their professional judgment, may disclose to a family member, other relative, close personal friend or any person you identify, PHI relevant to that person's involvement in your care or payment related to your care.

Health-related Personal communications: We may contact you to provide refill reminders or information about treatment alternatives or other health-related benefits and services that may be of interest to you.

Food and Drug Administration (FDA): We may disclose to the FDA, or persons under the jurisdiction of the FDA, its agents PHI relative to adverse events with respect to drugs, foods, supplements, products and product defects, or post marketing surveillance information to enable product recalls, repairs, or replacement.

Worker's compensation: We may disclose PHI about you as authorized by and as necessary to comply with laws relating to worker's compensation or similar programs established by law.

Public health: As required by law, we may disclose PHI about you to public health or legal authorities charged with preventing or controlling disease, injury, or disability.

Law enforcement: We may disclose PHI about you for law enforcement purposes as required by law or in response to a valid subpoena or other legal process.

As required by law: We must disclose PHI about you when required to do so by law.

Health oversight activities: We may disclose PHI about you to an oversight agency for activities authorized by law. These oversight activities include audits, investigations, and inspections, as necessary for our licensure and for the government to monitor the health care system, government programs, and compliance with civil rights laws.

Judicial and administrative proceedings: If you are involved in a lawsuit or a dispute, we may disclose PHI about you in response to a court or administrative order. We may also disclose PHI about you in response to a subpoena, discovery request, or other lawful process by someone else involved in the dispute, but only if efforts have been made to tell you about the request or to obtain an order protecting the requested PHI.

We are permitted to use or disclose PHI about you for the following purposes:

Research: We may disclose PHI about you to researchers when their research has been approved by an institutional review board that has reviewed the research proposal and established protocols to ensure the privacy of your information.

Coroners, medical examiners, and funeral directors: We may release PHI about you to a coroner or medical examiner. This may be necessary, for example, to identify a deceased person or determine the cause of death. We may also disclose PHI to funeral directors consistent with applicable law to carry out their duties.

Organ or tissue procurement organizations: Consistent with applicable law, we may disclose PHI about you to organ procurement organizations or other entities engaged in the procurement, banking, or transplantation of organs for the purpose of tissue donation and transplant.

Fundraising: We may contact you as part of a fundraising effort.

Notification: We may use or disclose PHI about you to notify or assist in notifying a family member, personal representative, or another person responsible for your care, your location, and your general condition.

Correctional institution: If you are or become an inmate of a correctional institution, we may disclose PHI to the institution or its agents when necessary for your health or the health and safety of others.

To avert a serious threat to health or safety: We may use and disclose PHI about you when necessary to prevent a serious threat to your health and safety or the health and safety of the public or another person.

Military and veterans: If you are a member of the armed forces, we may release PHI about you as required by military command authorities. We may also release PHI about foreign military personnel to the appropriate military authority.

National security and intelligence activities: We may release PHI about you to authorized federal officials for intelligence, counterintelligence, and other national security activities authorized by law.

Protective services for the President and others: We may disclose PHI about you to authorized federal official so they may provide protection to the President, other authorized persons or foreign heads of state or conduct special investigations.

Victims of abuse, neglect, or domestic violence: We may disclose PHI about you to a government authority, such as a social service or protective services agency, if we reasonably believe you are a victim of abuse, neglect, or domestic violence. We will only disclose this type of information to the extent required by law, if you agree to the disclosure, or if the disclosure is allowed by law and we believe it is necessary to prevent serious harm to you or someone else or the law enforcement or public official that is to receive the report represents that it is necessary and will not be used against you.

Other Uses and Disclosures of PHI
The Pharmacy will obtain your written authorization before using or disclosing PHI about you for purposes other than those provided for above (or as otherwise permitted or required by law). You may revoke this authorization in writing at any time. Upon receipt of the written revocation, we will stop using or disclosing PHI about you, except to the extent that we have already taken action in reliance on the authorization.

For More Information or to Report a Problem
If you have questions or would like additional information about the Pharmacy's privacy practices, you may contact the **[Privacy Officer]** at **[contact information].** If you believe your privacy rights have been violated, you can file a complaint with the **[Privacy Officer]** or with the Secretary of Health and Human Services. There will be no retaliation for filing a complaint.

Effective Date
This Notice is effective as of **[publication date].**

SELF-ASSESSMENT QUESTIONS CHAPTER VII

1. Acknowledgement signatures from patients
   a. are needed before a pharmacist can fill a prescription
   b. must be collected utilizing a specific form designed by the Department of Health and Human Services
   c. can be collected in a variety of ways including electronically
   d. None of the above

2. The rule "minimum necessary" as used in this chapter refers to:
   a. the least amount of medication that should be dispensed at any one time
   b. providing the least amount of protected health information as necessary to complete the task at hand
   c. the least amount of money a patient should be charged for pharmacy services provided
   d. None of the above

3. Under the privacy rule patients have a right to:
   a. Access their protected health information (PHI)
   b. Request that they be contacted at work, rather than at home for confidential reasons
   c. Both (a) and (b) are correct
   d. None of the above

4. The penalties under the HIPAA privacy rule
   a. provide for civil and criminal penalties that include both fines and jail time
   b. only pertain to the pharmacy and not the individual
   c. are enforced by the American Civil Liberties Union (ACLU)
   d. None of the above

5. Which of the following statements regarding HIPAA privacy rule is **false**?
   a. A pharmacy may deny a patient's request to amend their PHI
   b. Incidental disclosures occur every time PHI is accidentally disclosed to someone other than the patient
   c. Under the privacy rule it is up to the pharmacist to use professional judgment before disclosing PHI to a caregiver
   d. Under HIPAA, an employee cannot be penalized criminally for violating the Privacy Rule

Answers:
1) c
2) b
3) c
4) a
5) d

PHARMACY TECHNICIAN COMPETENCY ASSESSMENT

Chapter VII

Description of Ability or Skill	Initials		Training Completed	
	Tech	R.Ph.	Date	Remarks
The technician trainee understands the main concepts of the federal privacy rules that impact on the technician's role.				
The technician trainee can describe certain procedures that must be followed during the dispensing process to comply with the privacy regulations.				
The technician trainee can communicate with patients and health care professionals in compliance with the privacy rules.				
The technician trainee can effectively maintain privacy when communicating with those other than the patient.				
The technician trainee understands the basic patient rights as described in the privacy regulations which may affect the technician's role.				

Chapter VIII

The Dispensing Process

EDUCATIONAL OBJECTIVES

After studying the material in this chapter, the technician trainee should be able to:

- Gather information missing from prescription forms
- Describe the purpose of patient profiles and how to enter, update, and maintain them
- Describe prescription information that will be entered into the computer
- Understand the compliance checks the pharmacy computer performs
- Take proper action when compliance alerts are given by the computer
- Use correct procedures to dispense prescriptions
- Describe the information conveyed on prescription labels and receipts
- Label products dispensed in original packages
- Use auxiliary labels
- Recognize the need to have a pharmacist check all work performed by a technician
- Describe the procedures that assure delivery of the correct prescriptions to patients
- Describe the time limits for refilling prescriptions
- File prescriptions properly

Important Note

Although this chapter discusses laws and regulations related to dispensing generic equivalents and requirements for prescription labels, it should be noted that these laws and regulations vary from state to state. For specific information about the requirements in your state, ask your pharmacist supervisor.

STEPS IN RECEIVING PRESCRIPTIONS

As a pharmacy technician, you are responsible for assisting pharmacists in dispensing new and refill prescriptions. The dispensing process begins with receiving the prescription. The three steps in receiving prescriptions are:

1. Verify that all information is legibly included on the prescription form.
2. Ask patients if they will wait for the prescription or return later.
3. Gather patient-specific information.

SUBURBAN ASSOCIATES, S.C.
2530 RIDGE ROAD   RICHMOND, VA 23227   804-264-8808

JAMES DOWNEY, M.D. AD2685610   RICHARD MCKENNA, M.D. AM5120693
PAMELA CONNELLY, M.D. AC2100903   GLORIA HALVERSON, M.D. AH2100903

NAME _George Reassner_   AGE _45_
ADDRESS _6154 Maple Lane_   DATE _4-2-07_

Rx

Naproxen 250 mg #60
Sig: ↑ p.o. bid for pain
and inflammation

Refill _1_ Times

MAY SUBSTITUTE _____ M.D.
MAY NOT SUBSTITUTE _G. Halverson_____ M.D.

An example of a prescription that is complete and legible.

Verify Information on the Prescription Form

The health and well-being of patients you serve depends upon your ability to accurately interpret the information on their prescriptions. This may be complicated by prescribers whose handwriting is difficult to read. Nevertheless, it is your responsibility to make sure all necessary information is legibly included on the prescription form. When you are given the prescription, you should first verify the spelling of the patient's name and the address. Next, verify the prescriber's name. If you cannot read the prescriber's name, ask the patient for the prescriber's name and print it legibly on the prescription form. However, never indicate that the prescription is difficult to read because patients may wonder if you can read the rest of it too!

If you cannot read a prescription, do not guess! Ask a pharmacist to interpret it. Pharmacists are never too busy to take the time to assure that patients receive the right medication. A pharmacist may be able to interpret the prescription based on experience with the prescriber's handwriting or familiarity with the medication, strength, or directions. You, too, will become more comfortable reading prescriptions as you gain experience.

Pharmacists never dispense prescriptions unless they are absolutely sure that everything is correct. If the handwriting cannot be read, they will call the prescriber to clarify the medication or instructions. Occasionally, prescribers make errors when writing a prescription. Computer programs and, most importantly, careful pharmacists should always catch such mistakes before the medication is dispensed. (The requirements for written prescriptions were listed in Chapter IV.)

Determine Whether Patients Will Wait

Ask patients (or their caregivers) if they will wait for the prescription or will return later. If they will return later, obtain an approximate time. If they wait, give them an estimate of the waiting time. In estimating waiting times, calculate about five minutes to fill each prescription ahead of the patient's.

Note: Do not underestimate the waiting time. Patients may be disappointed to learn that a 20-minute wait lies ahead of them. They will be even more irritated, however, if that 20 minutes becomes 35. Trying to appease patients by shortening estimated waiting times makes them more impatient. Overestimating is always safer than underestimating. If the wait will be long, it is better to prepare the patient. They can then decide to wait in the pharmacy department or return later.

Gather Patient-Specific Information

Below are examples of patient-specific information that you will need to gather while filling a prescription. You will need this information to update the electronic patient record in the pharmacy's computer system.

- **Ask for patients' dates of birth.** For new patients, note the birth date on the prescription form and then enter it into the patient profile. This information is especially important to help pharmacists verify dosages for young children. The birth date is also helpful to determine dosages for older patients and to verify third-party program eligibility for older children covered by their parents' health insurance.

- **Ask patients about any allergies to medications.** This information is important for pharmacists' evaluations of prescriptions. If patients have allergies to medications, note them on the prescription form and then enter them in their patient profile. If patients have no allergies to medication, write NKA (No Known Allergies) on the prescription form. This notation confirms that you have asked them the question.

- **Ask patients if any health conditions have developed since their last visit to the pharmacy department.** Again, this new diagnosis should be entered into the computer, when possible, so that it can become part of the drug-disease alert procedure.

- **Ask if patients are currently taking other medications.** This includes over-the-counter (OTC) medications, too. Here, you are obtaining information the pharmacist can use to check for drug interactions. When possible, enter it into the patient profile. This information prepares pharmacists to counsel patients.

- **Ask patients if they have third-party coverage.** Also determine whether their coverage has changed since their last visit to the pharmacy. This will prevent problems with third-party eligibility that may prevent you from completing the prescription data entry until you are able to talk with the patient again. Obtaining this information will save both you and the patient some time.

All these questions sound like there is a lot to remember—and there is. After you have been through the routine a few times, you will see how quickly these questions can be covered. After you get to know patients, you will not need to ask all of these questions each time.

STEPS IN THE DISPENSING/ PRESCRIPTION FILL PROCESS

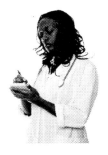

Prescription
written by authorized
prescriber.

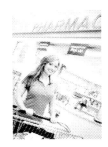

Patient or
representative presents
prescription to the
pharmacy.

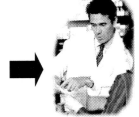

Prescription is checked
for completeness:
prescriber info, drug
name, strength, dose,
and directions.

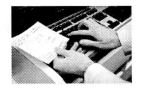

Correct patient info is
entered into computer
system.

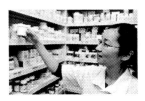

Prescription is prepared.
Correct amount of med prescribed
is measured and placed into
container.

Pharmacy Label is
generated. Make sure all the
legal items are identified.

Prescription is interpreted
and confirmed by pharmacy
system. Third party is billed
online.

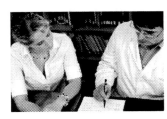

Prescription is prepared by
pharmacy technician, and final
check done by pharmacist.

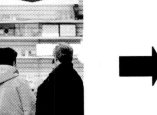

Patient or representative receives
script, pharmacy technician must
offer counseling to the patient. Then
script is rung on cash register, and
insurance log signed. Also HIPPA
form signed.

Pharmacist provides
counseling on the medication
prescribed and all medically
related questions.

After you receive a prescription and verify all the information, you begin to fill it. A brief outline of the procedure for filling a prescription is described below. Each step is described in detail.

Although the work flow or procedures in your pharmacy department may be carried out in a different order than the one given here, the basic principles still apply. Each step must be completed accurately. Pharmacists will establish routines to check your work to ensure everything is done correctly.

The steps in the dispensing process are:

1. Create or update patient profiles
2. Enter prescription information into the computer
3. Update files and print labels
4. Pull stock packages from the shelves
5. Check medication
6. Prepare medication
7. Have a pharmacist check your work
8. Bag the prescription

Create or Update Patient Profiles

In the pharmacy department, patients' records are referred to as "Patient profiles." Patient profiles provide valuable health care information that helps pharmacists ensure the proper use of prescription medications. Profiles also provide patients with records of expenditures on prescriptions and medical supplies that can be used for insurance records or income tax purposes. Patient profiles contain the following information:

- Demographic information (name, address, telephone numbers, date of birth, sex, etc.)
- Medication or prescription history
- Medication allergies
- Chronic conditions or diseases
- Third-party information

The medication history section of a patient profile also contains information about a prescription refill history. This history is useful for detecting compliance problems and for checking for drug interactions.

Selecting the correct profile for each patient is critical. If you cannot locate a patient's name in the computer, call the prescriber's office to obtain the information you need to identify the person correctly. If a prescriber telephones a prescription for a patient whose name is the same as others listed in the computer, ask the prescriber to verify to whom the prescription belongs or wait for the patient to come into the pharmacy department. In most instances, if two patients with the same name are in the computer, requesting the patient's address will identify the correct patient.

Enter Prescription Information into the Computer

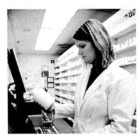

Become familiar with the procedure for entering prescription information into your pharmacy's computer system. If the prescription form is filled out properly, you will have most, if not all, of the information needed to complete or update a profile.

Select the prescriber. Following the directions provided for your computer system, choose the correct prescriber from the menu that appears on the computer screen.

Select the medication. Choose the correct medication, strength, dosage form, and package size. If generic medications are available, you may retrieve that generic from the area on the shelf where it is stored.

Many computers show a list of generic equivalents that can be substituted for the brand-name medication prescribed. When you enter a prescribed brand-name medication into the computer, it will tell you if it is a multiple-source medication and ask if you want to select a generic product. You may answer "yes" or "no" according to the prescriber's, patient's, or third-party payer's wishes, and according to state law. You must ask a pharmacist how to determine when to use generic products. (See chapter entitled, "Prescription Medication-Generics" for more information.)

If you answer "yes," the computer will show you a list of the manufacturers who make that medication in the prescribed strength and dosage form. Each will have its NDC number or order number listed with it. Other systems will only display one generic product for each brand, which makes selecting a generic medication easier. Also, remember to choose a product that you know is in stock.

> **Note:** In many states, only a pharmacist can choose which product can be substituted. Technicians should check with pharmacist with regard to state laws and regulations governing generic substitution.

Patient directions. Accurately interpreting prescribers' directions when entering them into the computer is very important. If you have any doubts about the prescriber's directions to the patient, or if you cannot read them, **ask a pharmacist to interpret them.** If you suspect that directions for use do not match the type of medication prescribed, a pharmacist should be notified immediately. The pharmacist may need to contact the prescriber for more information.

Although many health professionals inform patients how to take prescribed medications, patients may forget those instructions or they may not understand them. That is why providing easy-to-understand directions for use is important to patients.

Computer checks. Once all the necessary information has been entered into the computer, it will perform several checks designed to alert pharmacists to potential problems. If the patient is covered by a third-party program, the third party's computer will run similar checks when it receives claims electronically. The third party may then send an alert message back to the pharmacy's computer.

Most pharmacy computer systems help to ensure that the current prescription:

- Is not a medication to which the patient is allergic
- Will not conflict with other medications the patient is taking
- Will not cause a problem with other medical conditions the patient has
- Is not being refilled too early or too late
- Is not too low or high a dose
- Will not affect the fetus if the patient is pregnant

Whenever the computer alerts you to these or other potential problems (usually by a pop-up message on the screen and/or some type of alarm sound), **you must tell a pharmacist about it.** The pharmacist will then decide how to handle the alert. Often, the pharmacist will discuss the issue with the patient and/or the prescriber and agree on a course of action. Once this is done, you will follow one of two courses of action:

1. **Cancel the prescription.** If the prescriber selects a different medication you will cancel the current prescription and start over with the new one. If the prescriber decides not to give the patient a medication after all, you will simply return the prescription to a pharmacist who will then discuss the issue with the patient.

2. **Continue processing the prescription.** If the prescriber or the pharmacist determines that there is no potential problem for the patient in question, you or the pharmacist will override the alert. A message such as **"RPh-OK"** will often suffice, or **"MD-OK"** when the prescriber is contacted. The override notation will become part of the patient's permanent record.

Because of the importance and the frequency of occurrence, a discussion of a few of the more than 20 alerts follows:

- *Medication allergies.* Your computer is programmed to screen the patient's prescription against all known allergies the patient might have. For example, if patients tell you on their first visit that they are allergic to penicillin, this information would be input into the computer. If a few months later they bring in a prescription for amoxicillin (a type of penicillin), and you enter this medication into the computer, the computer will recognize that this patient is allergic to the prescribed product and will alert you to the potential problem. You will then handle the alert as outlined above.

- *Drug interactions.* Occasionally, the effect of a medication is changed by another medication that patients are taking at the same time. These "Drug interactions" are usually classified by their severity. If the computer indicates a potential drug interaction, you will handle the alert as outlined previously.

- *Contraindications.* When you initiate a profile for a new patient, it is important to note any chronic illnesses or diseases that the patient has. Some illnesses prevent people from taking certain medications, and serious reactions can occur if products are not prescribed carefully for these patients. If patients are taking prescribed medications that are not compatible with one of their diseases or chronic conditions (i.e., a contraindication), the computer may alert you. As with the other alert messages, a pharmacist will decide how to resolve the matter and you will handle the alert as outlined previously.

- *Early refill/overuse alert.* This check detects prescription refills that occur before the supply of the previous dispensing should have been completely used. There are many reasons this might occur:

  1. Patients' physicians may tell them to increase the dose of their medication after the last dispensing
  2. Patients may have come in for other refills and do not want to make another trip for the refill in question
  3. Patients may be going on vacation
  4. Patients may be taking more of the medication than has been prescribed

Before pharmacists override this alert or call the third party for an authorization to refill the prescription, they must determine why the refill is early. You can help pharmacists by tactfully discussing the timing of the refill with patients and then relaying that information. The pharmacist will then take the appropriate action.

Update Files and Print Labels

Update the computer. Once all the information from the prescription form is entered into the computer and the price of the prescription is calculated, enter your initials (or a pharmacist's) into the computer. Some states require both technicians and pharmacists to enter their initials. Check with a pharmacist to find out what is required both by the state and by the pharmacy department where you work.

This authorization, (typing in your initials, or having pharmacists type in theirs) signals the end of the prescription entry. The computer then automatically:

- Updates patient profiles and daily prescription logs
- Prints patient labels for prescription containers
- Prints prescription information labels (to be filed with original prescription forms in the pharmacy department)
- Prints patients' receipts

Additional information may be printed by the computer, such as patient information sheets prepared for the medication dispensed.

Labels for the prescription containers. Almost all the information required to be on labels that are affixed to prescription containers comes from original prescription forms. The following information is required on container labels:

- Pharmacy name, address, and telephone number
- Patient's name
- Dispensing Date
- Directions for use

- Prescription's serial number
- Prescriber's Name
- Medication's name, strength, and dosage form

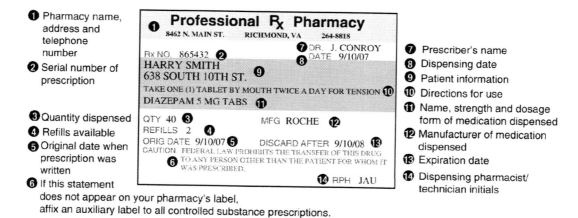

Information commonly printed on the prescription container label.

❶ Prescription number
❷ Retail price or co-pay
❸ Dispensing date and time
❹ Dispensing pharmacist/ technician initials
❺ Quantity dispensed
❻ Type of container cap
❼ Manufacturer
❽ Prescriber's DEA number and telephone
❾ Prescriber information

❿ Patient information
⓫ Medication information
⓬ Directions for use
⓭ Days supply (usually calculated by the computer)
⓮ Dispense As Written area indicates whether generic substitution is permissible or not. (Not filling this in indicates "yes.")

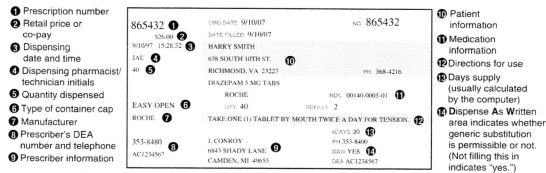

Prescription information label to be filed.

> **Note:** Some states require the quantity of the medication and/or its expiration date. Some states also require that both the brand and generic name of the medication appear on the label, as well as the number of refills available. Check with a pharmacist about your state's requirements.

Receipts. Receipts are affixed to the outside of prescription bags for clerks or cashiers to use when patients pick up their prescription. These labels generally include:

- Patient's name
- Medication name, strength, and dosage form
- Quantity dispensed
- Dispensing date
- Amount to be paid by the patient

❶ Pharmacy Information
❷ Patient Information
❸ Prescription Number
❹ Medication Information
❺ Quantity Dispensed
❻ Dispensing pharmacist/ technician initials
❼ Refills Remaining

❽ Type of Container Cap
❾ Dispensing Date
❿ Prescriber's Information
⓫ Retail Price or Co-payment

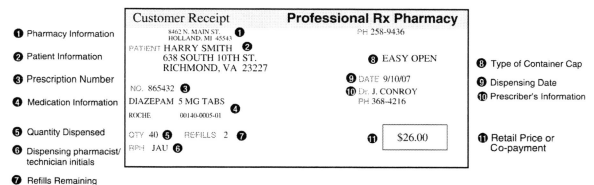

A receipt may be printed for the patient to submit for third-party reimbursement or tax purposes.

Additional information. Your computer may identify auxiliary labels that should be attached to prescription containers, or print medication information for patients. Collect all information printed by the computer for a pharmacist to check.

Pull Stock Packages from the Shelves

After labels are printed, find the stock bottle on the shelf. Confirm the spelling of the medication by comparing the stock bottle to the original prescription form. Check that the stock bottle contains enough tablets, capsules, liquid, etc. to fill the prescription. Even if you have used that bottle earlier in the day, you cannot be sure that another member of the staff has not depleted the supply since you last handled it.

Check your pharmacy's policy on what to do when there is not enough medication in stock to completely fill a prescription. The most important thing to remember, however, is that you should never tell patients to have their prescriptions filled at another pharmacy unless you are told by the pharmacist to do so.

There are several ways to handle out-of-stock situations. If there is some medication in the stock bottle, but not enough for the entire prescription, some pharmacies, for example, may dispense a few days' supply until the order arrives and they can dispense the rest. (For partial filling of controlled substances, see chapter entitled, "Controlled Substances".) When completely out-of-stock, some pharmacies notify patients immediately and schedule a later pick-up date. Check with a pharmacist to see how this is done in your pharmacy.

Check Medication

Always double-check to make sure you have selected the correct medication stock bottle. It is critically important to accurately identify the name, strength, and dosage form of the prescribed medication. A good checking process is to read the product label three times. Here is how to use this three-step check system:

1. When you go to the stock shelf, select the product, first by name. Verify the NDC number, for example, by matching what is shown on the computer screen with what is printed on the stock bottle label.

2. Check the label again before pouring or counting the medication to make sure you have selected the correct product and correct strength of the medication.

3. Before you present the prescription for a pharmacist to approve, check the stock bottle's label one more time.

With the eventual adoption of bar code technology, pharmacy computer systems will allow the pharmacist or technician to scan the stock bottle label to verify that the medication selected from the shelf matches the prescription record in the computer system.

As you remove the container from the stock shelf, check its expiration date. Make sure that you do not dispense medication that has expired or will expire before the patient uses it. If a medication's expiration date lists only month and year, the product will expire on the last day of that month, not the first day of the month. With the increased use of bar-code technology, pharmacists or technicians will be able to scan the stock bottle label to verify that the medication dispensed matches the prescription record in the computer system.

Prepare Medication

As you pour or count the product, check for any product defects such as broken tablets. These defects can occur during manufacture, shipping, and storage. If you have any doubts about a product's quality or stability, ask a pharmacist to check it.

Counting equipment and automated systems vary among pharmacy departments depending on the volume of prescriptions filled. Some pharmacy departments count tablets and capsules manually on counting trays; others have automatic counting machines that vary in design and complexity. Some are simple trays with holes in them through which you shake the dosage units. Others count dosage units via an electronic eye.

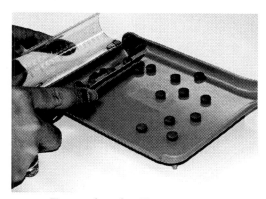

Example of a Counting Tray

Some sophisticated and costly machines store medications in large bins and count them automatically when the quantity to be dispensed is entered on a keypad or into the pharmacy computer. The machine interprets the prescription order, counts the proper number of dosage units, places them in the vial, prepares a label and affixes the label to the vial.

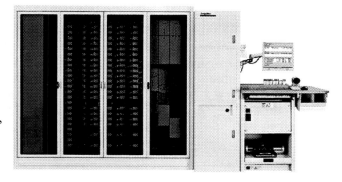

An example of the ScriptPro ® SP 200 ® Prescription Dispensing System.

These units require bulk drug products to be placed into individual bins. It is important that the bins be properly labeled with the name, strength and lot number of the medication. Some pharmacies also record the NDC number. For generic products, it is also a good idea to include the name of the manufacturer or distributor.

The pharmacy should have a policy and procedure manual that specifies the steps for filling the bins and verifying their accuracy. Since it is ultimately the pharmacist's responsibility to assure accuracy, the pharmacist should check any work done by a technician. Even though the prescription was prepared by the machine, it must still be checked by a pharmacist.

Automated systems were adopted in both hospital and community pharmacies to help improve inventory control and permit more effective use of personnel. Even more importantly, automated systems have helped to reduce dispensing errors. Pharmacy technicians are often given responsibilities for maintaining these automated systems. Technician duties may involve several manual functions such as: checking for expiration dates and stock outs, filling cells, logging lot numbers, cleaning cells, and keeping proper records. Technicians carefully document their work and all work is carefully checked by the pharmacist.

Since each pharmacy develops its own policies and procedures and designs its own workflow, it is important that you are thoroughly familiar with your own pharmacy's policies. If your pharmacy uses an automated system, be sure to carefully follow the pharmacy's policies and procedures. Patient safety depends upon strict adherence to these policies and procedures.

Note: When you use a counting tray or a counting machine, you will probably pour out more medication than you need. Before you pour the surplus back into the stock bottle, double-check its label to make sure you have the correct stock bottle.

Caution: Most pharmacy departments do not use automatic counting machines to count penicillin because many patients are allergic to this medication and the residue that remains in counting machines can contaminate future prescriptions. Penicillin is usually counted manually on a counting tray which is cleaned after filling the prescription.(Some pharmacies have separate trays used only for counting penicillin.)

After you have counted the medication, keep the vial, the computer-generated prescription label, auxiliary labels, any patient information pamphlets, and the stock container together until a pharmacist checks your work. Tighten the stock bottle cap securely to make sure that nobody pours a different medication into it. Replacing the cap securely protects the stock medication from moisture, light, and air. It also prevents you from spilling the product accidentally.

Dispensing liquid medications

Bottles. Whenever possible, select a bottle that holds exactly the amount of fluid you are dispensing. If you do not have the exact size, use the next larger size, but include an auxiliary label telling the patient that the bottle does contain the prescribed amount of medication.

Measuring with a graduate. For more accurate measurements, use a clean, dry, conical graduate or a graduated cylinder for measuring liquid medications. Both are referred to as "graduates." Conical graduates are easier to use when mixing two or more medications; graduated cylinders, on the other hand, are somewhat easier to use for measuring liquids accurately. After pouring the medication into the prescription bottle, compare the amount of medication to the markings on the bottle as a double check.

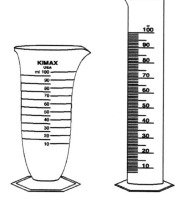

An example of a conical (left) and cylindrical graduate used for measuring liquid

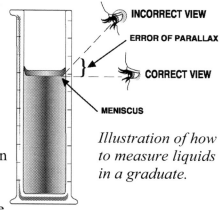

Illustration of how to measure liquids in a graduate.

- **Reading the meniscus.** When you pour a liquid into a graduate, it clings to the sides because of a force called "surface tension." This force causes the surface of the liquid to appear higher on the sides than in the center. This surface is called a "meniscus." To measure accurately, pour some of the liquid into the graduate then hold it at eye level and measure the liquid from **the bottom of the meniscus.** This will prevent a measurement error. If you pour too much liquid into the graduate, carefully pour the excess amount back into the stock bottle.

Note: You must shake some liquids before you measure them. The manufacturer's label will indicate whether the medication must be shaken.

- **Turn the label toward you.** Before you pour the medication from the stock bottle into the graduate or any other container, make sure the label of the stock bottle is turned up. This way, if you drip or spill any of the liquid, it will not ruin the label. Of course, if you do drip or spill the product, you should wipe off the container and any other soiled surfaces immediately with a damp paper towel or a cloth. Keep the neck of the stock bottle clean as well. Besides making the bottle look messy, dried liquid on the neck may leave a residue that causes the cap to stick to the container, making it hard to open next time. (This is true of prescription bottles, too.)

Reconstituting powders to liquids. Because of rapid deterioration, and because prescriptions are not always picked up right away, pharmacists may ask you to wait until patients are in the pharmacy department before reconstituting powders. If reconstituted products must be held for patients, be sure to label them with the expiration date and a notice to keep the medication refrigerated.

Before adding water to a powdered medication, loosen the powder by tapping the bottle a few times, or turn the bottle upside-down and hit it with the palm of your hand to loosen the powder from the bottom of the bottle. The amount of water you need to add is provided in metric units on the medication label.

Usually you pour about one-half of the water from the graduate or reconstituting tube into the prescription bottle. Put the cap on tightly and shake the bottle vigorously. Turn the bottle upside-down. Check to make sure that no powder is stuck to the bottom. If necessary, use a glass stirring rod to loosen any caked powder. Shake the bottle again. Add the remaining water and shake once more.

- **If you use a graduate,** fill it to the desired level with water. Hold the cylinder at eye level after you add the water and read the bottom of the meniscus. If you add too much water, pour some into the sink.

Note: All reconstituted preparations need the "Shake Well" auxiliary label. Most also need a "Keep in Refrigerator" label and another label showing an expiration date of 10 to 14 days from the reconstitution date.

Note: Use distilled water only—never use ordinary tap water. Distilled water prevents impurities and mineral salts from reacting with the medication. Measure water using either a graduate or reconstituting devices.

- **If you use a reconstituting tube,** which is a device that allows water to run into a graduated measuring tube, you will find it mounted on the wall at eye level under the water container. Before you use this device, make sure the clamp on the lower delivery tube is closed—an open tube will run a stream of water over the front of your pharmacy jacket, pants, skirt, or shoes. Make sure you close the clamp when you finish using the device.

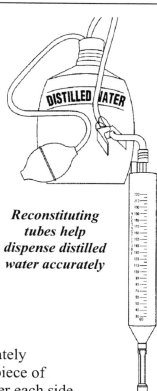

Reconstituting tubes help dispense distilled water accurately

> **Note:** Be careful! When you take off the cap or add water to powder, some of the dry material may blow into the air. If this happens, try not to inhale the powder. Many people are allergic to penicillin; others could develop allergies to other medications as well.

Labeling prescription containers. Once medications are appropriately packaged, lay the patient labels face up on the counter and place a piece of pharmacy tape over them so that a small amount of tape extends over each side. Pick up the tape (with label attached) and place the label neatly on the container.

If the label has a self-stick backing, try another approach. Lay the container down on the counter and neatly affix the label horizontally, using both hands. Cover the label with tape. Be careful not to leave fingerprints on the label or the tape.

Labels for products in original packages. There are a number of prescription medications that are supplied to the pharmacy department in original packages. These products do not need to be counted, poured, or processed in any way by pharmacy personnel—they are dispensed to the patient as is. Some examples are:

- Nitroglycerin tablets
- Topical ointments and creams
- Metered dose inhalers
- Eye and ear medication
- Suppositories
- Transdermal patches
- Oral contraceptives

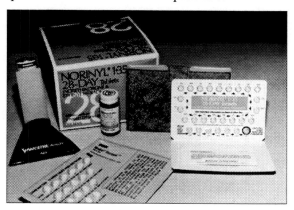

Examples of medications dispensed in their original packages.

These products, however, must still be labeled correctly before they can be given to patients. Since most packages have directions for use and other important information printed on them, be careful where you place labels. If possible, put labels directly on the container that patients will use (i.e., on the glass bottle, ointment tube, inhaler device, or plastic case containing oral contraceptives, etc.) If the container is too small for a label to fit, you have two options:

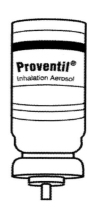

1. Carefully trim the label and put it on the bottle or tube.

2. Package the bottle or tube containing the medication into its original box or a plastic vial. Put the label on the box or vial. You should also put a small label with the pharmacy department's name, prescription number, patient's name, and prescriber's name on the original package. If a label is put on a box, there are usually two sides of the box that have little or no printing on them; this is a good place to put the label.

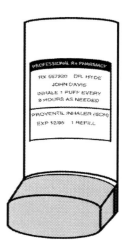

Adding Auxiliary Labels. Auxiliary labels convey additional instructions to patients:

- How and when to take medication
- What foods or medications to avoid while taking the medication
- How to store the medication
- How to administer the medication
- What side effects can occur
- Number of refills remaining
- When the medicine expires

An example of a properly labeled inhaler

Auxiliary labels are usually colorful to attract patients' attention and to make it easier for you to distinguish between the labels as you select them. If your computer system cannot indicate which auxiliary labels to use, ask a pharmacist to identify labels to accompany specific medications.

Auxiliary labels should be placed neatly on the prescription bottle. They should not cover any information on patient labels.

Twenty Commonly Used Warning Labels

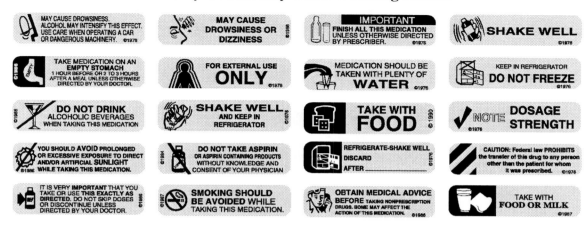

Pharmex Copyrighted Warning Labels were reprinted with authorization by TimeMed Labeling Systems, Inc.

A commonly-used auxiliary label for reconstituted antibiotics reminds the patient: "Refrigerate; Shake Well; Discard this medicine after: _____" The date entered is usually 10 to 14 days after the reconstitution date.

Controlled substances in Schedules II through IV are required to have the following notice on the prescription label or on an auxiliary label that says: "Caution: Federal law prohibits transfer of this drug to any person other than the patient for whom it was prescribed."

Include patient information. Pharmaceutical manufacturers sometimes supply information written specifically for patients about a medication's use and its potential side effects. Your pharmacy may also have a system for generating a patient information leaflet or sheet.

Have a Pharmacist Check Your Work

Pharmacists have different procedures for preparing prescriptions and different ways of checking a technician's work. Your job as a technician is to assist pharmacists. The final responsibility for the accuracy of the prescription, however, rests with them. Pharmacists must always check prescriptions before they are dispensed to patients to insure that the container:

- Has the correct medication
- For the correct patient
- In the correct dose and strength
- For the correct route of administration
- With the correct directions

When conducting the final check, some pharmacists want technicians to put the medication in the prescription container, label the container and leave it on the counter along with the original prescription form, the medication's stock bottle, and the receipt. Other pharmacists ask that you do not attach the prescription label and auxiliary labels to the containers. They prefer, or are required (depending on state law), to check the prescription and attach the label themselves.

Preparing Prescription for Pick-up

After pharmacists have checked and approved prescriptions, put containers and any patient information sheets in bags and staple the receipts on the outside or place the receipts in the bags. (Check with a pharmacist as to policy or preference.) Whenever possible, put all prescriptions dispensed to patients at the same time into one bag. It is easy to mix up the bottles and bags if there are several prescriptions being filled at the same time.

If patients do not wait in the pharmacy department for the prescription, put the bag into the holding bin. Most pharmacy departments have bins that allow you to store prescriptions in alphabetical order by last name.

If patients have not picked up a prescription they requested at an earlier date, make sure that they still need the prescription. Prescribers may have discontinued a patient's medication and replaced it with another prescription.

Duties at the "Out Window"

If the patient is waiting, say, "Ms. Newman, your prescription is ready." If the patient is shopping in the aisles, announce, "Ms. Newman, your prescription is ready. Please return to the pharmacy department." If the patient does not answer your page, alphabetically file the prescription in the completed prescription area for later pick-up.

Right medication to the right patient. When patients return to pick up their medications, you should verify that they receive the correct prescription. A suggested procedure is outlined below:

- **Verify the number of prescriptions being picked up.** Prescriptions may have been bagged separately during the filling process.

- **Check the prescription.** Whenever you bag prescriptions for later pick-up or ring the sale immediately, always compare the prescription number and the patients' names on the prescription packages to the numbers and names on the prescription labels. You may have more than one patient with a common name, like Davis or Williams. Double-checking receipts and labels avoids giving the wrong medication to the wrong person.

- **Check the receipt for any third-party notations.** Remember, if the patient presents you with a third-party card, you will collect from the patient only the amount of copayment the patient owes.

- **Inform patients that a pharmacist will be glad to discuss their medication with them or answer any questions they have.** Inform a pharmacist immediately if patients have questions. In some cases, pharmacists will indicate that they want to see particular patients when they pick up their prescriptions. In this case, politely tell patients that a pharmacist will be with them in a moment to discuss their medication. (Some states require the pharmacist to counsel every patient, so check with the pharmacist regarding your state's practice regulations.)

- **Process the sale by following normal cash register procedures and finish the transaction in your usual friendly manner.** Thank patients and encourage them to call a pharmacist if they have any questions later about the medication.

Signature logs. Patients are sometimes required to sign a log documenting that they have made particular transactions. Signature logs are used for purchases of Medicaid and other third-party prescriptions, Schedule V over-the-counter medications, and hypodermic needles and syringes.

- **Third-party signature log.** Most third-party programs require patients to sign a third-party signature log to document that they have received the medication. All information entered into the log is usually found on the prescription receipt. Some pharmacies request Medicaid patients to sign an additional section of the log, documenting that pharmacists have offered to counsel them about using their medications.

- **Schedule V sales record log.** The sale of OTC Schedule V items are recorded in a Schedule V sales record log, kept at the register in the pharmacy department. (See chapter entitled, "Controlled Substances-Schedule V Records Log".)

- **Poisons.** The sale of some poisons requires a record of the date of sale, the name and address of the purchaser, the name and quantity of the poison, and the purpose of the purchase. Usually this log is kept near the register.

- **Needles and syringes.** In some states, the purchase of needles and syringes must be recorded in a log signed by the patient.

Refills

Refill procedures. Patients may call in refill requests by telephone or come by in person. Often patients bring empty containers or prescription receipts, making your job much easier. You can simply enter the prescription number into the computer and call up all the information you need.

If patients do not have containers or receipts or do not know the name of their medication, ask these questions: "What is the medication for?" "What size and color is it?" Work with a pharmacist to determine exactly which medication is to be refilled; then, verify the medication's appearance with the patients.

Refill the prescription just as you would an original prescription. Keep in mind, however, that it is easy for patients to make mistakes when reading or writing down prescription numbers for a refill. When you enter the prescription number into the computer, make sure you fill the correct prescription for the correct patient and verify the patient's name and address. If the patient brings in an empty container or a prescription receipt, make sure the information that appears on the computer screen or in the file matches that on the container or receipt.

Some states also require a pharmacy technician and a pharmacist to initial the back of the prescription form, adding the date of renewal and the quantity dispensed (if this information is different than what appears on the face of the prescription). When a pharmacist's initials and the date of refill are the only items recorded on the back of the prescription form, it is assumed that the refill was for the full amount of the prescription order. Pharmacy departments that are computerized may meet this requirement by printing out a daily log of prescriptions dispensed and having the pharmacist(s) who dispensed the prescriptions sign the log.

The computer will automatically decrease the number of remaining refills when the prescription is processed. If this information is not automatically printed on the prescription label, put an auxiliary label on the prescription bottle to remind patients how many refills remain.

Refill regulations. By law, prescriptions may only be refilled if prescribers authorize them. Usually prescribers mark the "Refill" space on the prescription form. However, sometimes prescribers indicate elsewhere on the prescription form that refills are permitted. If the number of refills is not indicated, physicians must be contacted for this information before the prescription can be refilled.

Be alert when reading refill information. If prescribers write "2" in the refill space, the prescription may be filled a total of three times, the original dispensing, plus two refills.

- **PRN refills.** PRN is a Latin abbreviation that means "as needed." PRN refills are allowed on prescription medications, usually for a maximum of one year. The total number of refills a patient may request will vary. Most states require a new prescription for PRN medications after one year. Check with a pharmacist to find out your state's requirements for PRN refills.

- **Controlled substances.** As described in the chapter entitled "Controlled Substances", Schedule II medications may not be refilled. Schedule III or IV medications cannot be refilled more than five times, or after six months of date of issue. Consult patient profiles when you receive a refill request for a Schedule III or IV medication to check that patients are not taking the controlled substance more frequently than prescribed.

- **Third-party prescriptions.** Many third-party policies limit the number of doses that may be dispensed at one time to a one-month's supply except for certain "maintenance medications," which may be dispensed in larger quantities. (This is discussed under the chapter entitled, "Managed Care Prescriptions".*)*

Recordkeeping

To assure that pharmacy department records are accurate, certain procedures must be followed each day. You may be asked to take care of all or some of them.

Original prescription forms. Even if your pharmacy department is computerized, you must still file original prescriptions by hand in numerical order. Note, however, that there are specific requirements for filing controlled-substance prescriptions, as described in chapter entitled, "Controlled Substances". As a result, the files must be orderly and organized so that written prescriptions can be easily retrieved to verify information such as date of issue, strength of medication, or number of refills. Filing original prescription forms may be one of your jobs. File prescriptions according to their prescription serial numbers. Most pharmacy departments bundle them in groups of 100.

Computer back-up. Many pharmacy departments back up the information from their computers on disk, tape, or some other type of electronic medium. This ensures that little or no information will be lost if the computer malfunctions. Usually a pharmacist takes care of this.

Daily log. Many pharmacies print out a hard copy (a paper record) of all new and refill prescriptions dispensed each day. This hard copy printout usually contains the following information about every prescription:

- The serial number of the prescription
- Dispensing date
- Patient's name
- Prescriber's name
- Medication name, strength and dosage form
- Quantity dispensed
- Initials or identification code of the dispensing pharmacist and/or technician

If the following information is not immediately retrievable on the computer screen, it, too, may have to be included on the daily printout:

- Patient's address
- Prescriber's address
- Prescriber's DEA number, provided prescription is for a controlled substance
- Quantity prescribed, if different from quantity dispensed
- Date of issue of the prescription, if it is different from the date of dispensing
- Total number of refills for that prescription dispensed to date

Instead of a hard-copy list of each day's new and refill prescriptions, some states require pharmacists to sign a statement or log attesting that the information entered into the computer for each prescription has been reviewed and is correct. These records are filed and kept in the pharmacy department for two to five years. You may be asked to prepare the printout and/or file the report.

SELF-ASSESSMENT QUESTIONS CHAPTER VIII

1. Pharmacy computer systems perform a number of checks to alert pharmacists to potential problems. Which of the following is generally NOT detected by the computer?
   a. Prescription is being refilled too early.
   b. Patient is allergic to a prescribed medication.
   c. Directions on prescription are incorrect.
   d. Medication causes a problem with patient's disease state.

2. To dispense 100 mL of a liquid medication, you should use as:
   a. 1-ounce bottle.
   b. 2-ounce bottle.
   c. 4-ounce bottle.
   d. 6-ounce bottle.

3. A contraindication is a:
   a. Direction by a pharmacist or physician that the patient should stop taking a certain prescription medication.
   b. Computer alert indicating that the patient is getting a prescription too soon.
   c. Situation in which the effect of one medication is changed by another medication that a patient is taking at the same time.
   d. Symptom or medical condition which indicates the inappropriateness of a form of treatment that would otherwise be advisable.

4. A prescription label must contain:
   a. The patient's address.
   b. The pharmacy's address.
   c. The prescriber's address.
   d. The date the physician wrote the prescription.

5. Reconstituted products:
   a. Must have a "shake well" label.
   b. Are usually reconstituted with tap water.
   c. Must have a "keep refrigerated" label.
   d. Are often reconstituted when placed on the shelf so they will be ready when a prescription is received.

Answers:
1) c
2) c
3) d
4) b
5) a

PHARMACY TECHNICIAN COMPETENCY ASSESSMENT
CHAPTER VIII

Description of Ability or Skill	Initials		Training Completed	
	Tech	R.Ph.	Date	Remarks
The technician trainee can describe what information is required on completed prescription forms and how to gather any information that might be missing.				
The technician trainee can describe the purpose of patient profiles and how to enter, update, and maintain them.				
The technician trainee successfully enters prescription information into the computer.				
The technician trainee is aware of the compliance/interaction checks the pharmacy computer performs.				
The technician trainee takes proper action when a compliance alert is noted when entering a prescription.				
The technician trainee uses correct procedures in preparing prescriptions for dispensing.				
The technician trainee can describe the different types of information conveyed on prescription labels and receipts.				

PHARMACY TECHNICIAN COMPETENCY ASSESSMENT
CHAPTER VIII
(Continued)

| Description of Ability or Skill | Initials | | Training Completed | |
	Tech	R.Ph.	Date	Remarks
The technician trainee can properly label products dispensed in original packages.				
The technician trainee properly uses auxiliary labels.				
The technician trainee understands the necessity of having a pharmacist check all work performed by the technician.				
The technician trainee use proper procedure to assure delivery of the correct prescriptions to patients.				
The technician trainee understands and can cite rules and regulations regarding time limits for refilling prescriptions.				
The technician trainee properly files prescriptions.				

Chapter IX
Managed Care Prescriptions

EDUCATIONAL OBJECTIVES

After studying the material in this chapter, the technician trainee should be able to:

- Differentiate among the various types of managed care prescription programs
- Describe the purpose of the various types of managed care prescription program coverage limitations
- Describe the three components of prescription reimbursement
- Explain the purpose of patient cost sharing and differentiate among various types
- Identify and prevent data-entry errors in managed care prescription claims
- Resolve problems with claims adjudication and reconciliation
- Understand the use of manual or electronic prescription signature logs

Over 85% of all prescriptions are paid by third-party programs. The term "third-party program" refers to both private health benefit programs and government programs that pay for prescriptions on behalf of patients. The term stems from the three parties involved:

1. The **patient** who receives the prescription
2. The **pharmacist** who dispenses the prescription
3. The **payer** who pays for all, or part, of the prescription

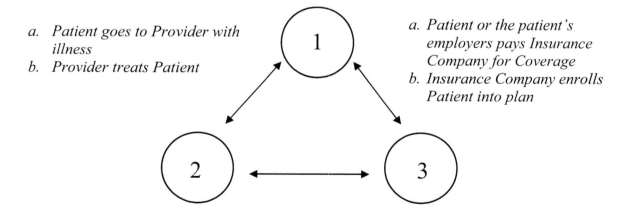

TYPES OF THIRD-PARTY PLANS

There are hundreds of third-party programs covering prescriptions in the United States. These programs can be classified in many ways, including:

- Degree of program management (i.e., traditional third-party plans or managed care programs)
- Type of program sponsor (i.e., public or private)

Degree of Program Management

The way in which a health insurance plan is organized and operates has a major impact on the degree of control it exercises over health care providers and, consequently, provider revenues and services. For the sake of simplicity, this chapter discusses three basic types of health insurance programs with an emphasis on the one type that now dominates the industry.

1. *Traditional indemnity.* These plans do not contract with health care providers and have little or no control over the utilization and cost of health care services. Patients pay the provider for each service provided (i.e., "fee-for-service" reimbursement) and submit their own claims to the insurance company for reimbursement. Although these plans were popular from the 1950s to the 1970s, they are not used much any more.

2. *Managed indemnity.* This type of health insurance includes plans that allow any provider to participate and reimburse on a discounted fee-for-service basis. Since the provider group is not restricted, these plans have limited ability to extract large volume discounts from providers. Patient cost sharing and some controls on utilization are also employed.

   For example, this means that the patient can choose the doctor that they would like to visit, but their health insurance may only pay a certain portion of the charges for the services that doctor provides to the patient. The patient may also have to pay the physician for the difference between what the health insurance plan pays and what the physician charged for a particular visit.

3. *Managed care.* The defining feature of these plans is the use of provider networks. These plans include or exclude providers based on their compatibility with the plan's objectives. There are several types of managed care organizations (MCOs) that are usually categorized based on their relationship with physicians. The two major types of MCOs are health maintenance organizations (HMOs) and preferred provider organizations (PPOs). The major difference between these two types of organizations is that HMOs make physicians assume some of the financial risk and generally restrict patients from using providers who are not part of the network. For example, if an individual has HMO coverage, the individual must see and use only "network" doctors.

PPOs, on the other hand, reimburse on a discounted fee-for-service basis but do cover some expenses for "non-participating providers" who are not part of the network. Patients pay a smaller percentage of the cost when they use a network – or "preferred"– provider. For example, a patient may pay a $10 copayment when visiting a network physician and $25 when visiting a non-preferred provider. An individual who has PPO coverage has the choice of physicians to visit; however, the individual may pay more if he/she chooses a doctor who is classified as an "out-of-network" provider.

Although HMOs generally control providers more than PPOs do, the various types of HMOs can vary widely in the amount of control they exercise.

Due to the complexities of administering and managing pharmacy benefits, MCOs often carve out prescription benefits and arrange to have them managed by organizations known as "pharmacy benefit managers" (PBMs). The administrative services provided by PBMs include:

- Contracting with pharmacies to provide specified services
- Communicating with both patients and providers to explain and update administrative policies
- Providing reports to plan sponsors
- Identifying eligible beneficiaries and issuing identification cards
- Processing claims submitted by pharmacies
- Reimbursing pharmacies
- Auditing pharmacies
- Controlling benefit use
- Ensuring program quality

PBMs enroll pharmacies with a "participating pharmacy agreement," a contract that stipulates the pharmacy services that will be provided in exchange for a specified reimbursement. The network of participating pharmacies may be an "open panel," in which all community pharmacies are invited to sign participating pharmacy agreements, or it may be a "closed panel," in which only selected or "preferred" pharmacies may participate. These preferred pharmacies often accept a lower reimbursement in anticipation of a greater number of patients.

Patients covered by managed care plans in which your pharmacy does not participate will need to pay cash for the prescription at the time of sale and then submit a claim form themselves to the plan for reimbursement. MCOs usually will not pay claims to non-participating pharmacies. You may be asked to fill out the pharmacy portion of the form. This sometimes happens with out-of-town patients visiting your community who need to have prescriptions filled.

Types of Program Sponsors

There are two major types of managed care prescription program sponsors:

- **Government agencies.** The two largest government programs are Medicaid and Medicare. Medicaid is administered by each state with partial funding from the federal government. Each state establishes its own income-based eligibility criteria for patients. Although prescription drug coverage is optional, each state Medicaid program currently covers prescription medications. Medicaid accounts for more than one out of every ten prescriptions. Since Medicaid programs are designed individually by the states, program coverage varies from state to state.

  Medicare, which provides health insurance for the aged and disabled, began covering outpatient prescription drugs in 2006 through Medicare Part D in an effort to make prescription drugs more affordable for covered individuals. The program is voluntary and requires beneficiaries to pay premiums plus share some of the costs for services. These premiums are reduced for low-income beneficiaries. To participate, eligible patients must enroll during limited enrollment periods. They have incentives to enroll early because they are charged higher costs if they delay enrollment. Certain patients who were eligible for both Medicare and Medicaid (known as "dual eligibles") now receive their prescription benefits through Medicare. The specifics of Medicare Part D plans vary from insure to insurer, but every participating health care plan must offer benefits that are financially equivalent, if not better than the "Standard Plan."

  The "Standard Plan" requires patients to pay a monthly premium and a deductible before Medicare covers any of their prescription costs. In 2006 the monthly premium was $35 and the deductible was $250. These amounts have been indexed annually. When patients' out-of-pocket costs exceed a specified amount ($2,500 in 2006) coverage actually stops until they spend enough for the coverage to start again. In 2006, patients had a coverage gap, known as the "donut hole," between $2,250 and $3,600 in out-of-pocket costs. Out-of-pocket costs are expected to rise as Medicare prescription expenditures rise. Therefore, the amounts for this "donut hole" are likely to change in future years. Once patients have expenditures exceeding the "donut hole" their coverage is reinstated with their insurance provider paying 95% of drug costs, leaving the patient to pay only 5%. The schedule resets once the calendar year has been completed.

  Insurance companies providing Medicare Part D coverage are free to make certain alterations to the Standard Plan, so premiums and out-of-pocket expenditures can vary significantly from one insurance carrier to another.

  Patients should be encouraged to do their own research prior to enrolling in any plans. There are a number of national and state plans that are available, but patients must realize that not all of them are the same. They must complete their own investigations into the parameters of each one and select the plan that best fits their needs.

Pharmacy technicians are likely to encounter situations where patients are confused about what is covered by their Medicare plan and what they must pay themselves. For example, they may have to pay 100% of their costs at first, then only 25% after they meet their deductible. Later in the year they may hit the donut hole and have to pay 100% of their costs again. Even later in the year, their coverage may be restored and they only have to pay 5% of the costs. Complicating this even more is the fact that their coverage may not be the same as that of their friends and relatives. Pharmacy technicians must be able to deal with these situations tactfully and patiently and answer questions while encouraging patients to become familiar with the requirements of their own individual plans.

Dual eligible recipients who have been switched from Medicaid to Medicare may also find that medications that were covered under Medicaid are no longer covered by their Medicare plan. Patients who have concerns about the change in their medication may need to be reassured that the medication they are receiving is the medication that was authorized. Be sure to refer any patient concerns that you cannot handle to the pharmacist or the individual in your pharmacy who is responsible for resolving prescription insurance problems.

- **Private insurance.** Most non-governmental managed care prescription programs are part of group health benefit plans offered to employees and their families by employer groups.

PRESCRIPTION REIMBURSEMENT

Reimbursement to pharmacies is typically based on payment for the drug ingredient cost plus a dispensing fee. A portion of the total cost is usually paid by the patient. The patient's out-of-pocket payment is known as "Patient cost sharing." A description of the three components of prescription reimbursement follows:

- **Drug ingredient cost** refers to the price the pharmacy department pays for the medication. For single-source medications (i.e., products without generic equivalents), MCOs usually base reimbursement for drug ingredient costs on a percentage of the drug product's published list price, also known as its "average wholesale price" (AWP) or the Wholesale Acquisition Cost (WAC). For example, a PBM may reimburse pharmacies for drug ingredient costs at 90 percent of AWP. Reimbursement for multiple-source medications, on the other hand, is often based on the MCO's "maximum allowable cost" (MAC), which is an estimate of the cost of a generic equivalent. Unless the physician orders a particular brand to be dispensed for medical reasons, pharmacists will choose to dispense a generically equivalent drug product and will only be paid the MAC. Often patients who choose to receive the brand are required to pay the difference between the brand price and MAC price.

> **Note:** At the time of this writing, it is expected that AWP will be replaced with a new measure known as Average Manufacturer's Price (AMP). This may significantly alter the amount that pharmacies are reimbursed for prescription drugs dispensed to Medicaid and/or Medicare patients.

- **Dispensing fees** are paid to cover the pharmacy department staff's labor and overhead expenses to fill the prescription and allow for a reasonable return on investment. There is continuing debate about the adequacy of such fees.

Sample Problem 1: Reimbursement

Assume that your pharmacy participates in XYZ Pharmacy Benefit Management Program and they will reimburse the pharmacy for brand-name drugs at AWP minus 15% plus a dispensing fee of $3.00. Calculate the reimbursement for the following prescription:

> Rx: Germacillin 250 mg.
> Sig: i cap bid
> Disp #20
> The AWP for the prescription is $86.00

Answer:

Reimbursement = (AWP – 15%) + $3.00
= ($86.00 – ($86.00 x 0.15) + $3.00
= ($86.00 -$12.90) + $3.00
= $73.10 + $3.00
= $76.10

OR

= ($86.00 x (1.0 – 0.15)) + $3.00
= ($86.00 x 0.85) + $3.00
= $73.10 + $3.00
= $76.10

- **Patient cost sharing** is designed to make patients more cost conscious and usually take the form of copayment, or deductibles and coinsurance.

1. **Copayments,** the most common form of patient cost sharing for prescription drugs, require patients to pay a specified dollar amount for every prescription received (e.g., $10.00 per prescription). Some managed care plans use tiered copayments that are lower for generic or preferred drug products and higher for brand-name or non-preferred drug products. Two, three and four-tier plans are common.

2. **Deductibles** require patients to pay for all of their prescription expenses until a specified dollar amount has been paid out-of-pocket. For example, the prescription plan may cover prescriptions only after the patient has paid the first $200 of prescription expenses.

3. **Coinsurance** is a form of patient cost sharing in which patients pay a specified percentage of their prescription expenses. For example, the MCO pays 80 percent of prescription costs and patients pay the remaining 20 percent. Until recently, coinsurance was infrequently used by PBMs. Now, however, several PBMs are starting to use it – especially in conjunction with tiered cost-sharing arrangements that impose a 50% coinsurance on the highest tier (usually called "lifestyle drugs"). It is expected that the use of coinsurance will continue to grow because it makes patients more sensitive to drug cost than copayments.

You will be expected to collect the patient's share of the prescription cost at the time the prescription is dispensed; this amount is then deducted from the managed care plan's reimbursement. It is important that you know the amount to collect. You should also be prepared to explain that the amount of cost sharing often varies depending upon the particular product that the physician prescribes and the plan's benefit design.

Sample Problem 2: Patient Cost Sharing

Using the example in Sample Problem 1 above, calculate the amounts to be paid by both XYZ Pharmacy Benefit Management Program and the patient in each of the following cases:

A) The patient must pay a $25.00 copayment.

B) The patient has a $200 deductible and a $25.00 copayment but has not received any other prescriptions yet this year.

C) The patient has a $200 deductible and a $25.00 copayment but already received other prescriptions this year totaling $350.

D) The patient has to pay a 20% coinsurance.

Answers:

A) Patient's co-payment is $25.00. PBM reimbursement to the pharmacy is $51.10 ($76.10 -$25.00)

B) Patient's responsibility (deductible) is $76.10. PBM will not reimburse the pharmacy

C) Patient's deductible is already met but patient must pay copayment of $25.00. PBM reimbursement to the pharmacy is $51.10

D) Patient's responsibility is $15.22 ($76.10 x 0.2). PBM reimbursement to the pharmacy is $60.88 ($76.10 x 0.8)

PROCESS FOR DISPENSING THIRD-PARTY PRESCRIPTIONS AND SUBMITTING CLAIMS

As third-party prescription volume continues to grow, it is increasingly important for pharmacy managers to establish standard policies and procedures for handling these prescriptions. To reduce the number of rejected claims or delayed claims payments, pharmacy staff members should know how to:

- Check patient eligibility
- Determine whether there are coverage limitations (e.g., restrictions on coverage of certain medications or quantities)
- Collect copayments and keep track of deductibles
- Submit claims to the correct insurance company
- Some of these issues are discussed in more depth in this chapter.

Eligibility

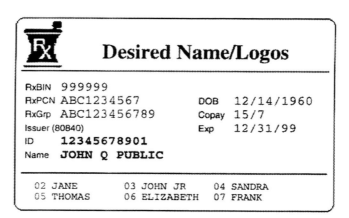

Example of a patient's third-party prescription identification card.

The participating pharmacy agreement specifies how covered employees and dependents will be identified. Although the PBM usually issues identification cards, these cards are difficult to retrieve when employees terminate employment and, therefore, cannot always be relied upon when determining eligibility. Pharmacies are usually required to verify patient eligibility through the pharmacy computer in a process known as "on-line adjudication."

Some plans' identification cards list the names of the cardholder and all dependents eligible to receive prescriptions. Other plans do not list eligible family members; instead, they define eligibility coverage. For example, dependent children may be covered up to age 18 or, in other cases, they may be covered up to age 23 or 24 (depending on the specific plan) if they are full-time students, etc.

Just as you will learn to recognize certain ID cards, you will also learn the exclusions and restrictions of many plans your pharmacy department accepts. Be familiar with your pharmacy's process for determining eligibility and benefit coverage limitations and exclusions and the procedures for entering information into the computer to satisfy data requirements.

If you are presented an unfamiliar identification card, follow the procedures established by your pharmacy. It may require you to call the PBM's help desk or review the pharmacy procedures manual. Always check with your pharmacist supervisor on how to handle these situations.

Submitting Claims

When prescription claims are received by PBMs they are first screened to make sure that they are complete, accurate, and consistent with contract requirements. Favorable adjudication requires that claims be submitted properly.

Pharmacies submit almost all claims electronically via the pharmacy computer system while the prescription is being dispensed. By linking pharmacies to PBMs at the time a prescription is dispensed, these "point-of-sale" (POS) systems help you to do the following:

- Verify that the patient is eligible for coverage
- Determine whether the prescribed medication is covered
- Determine whether there is a maximum allowable cost for multiple source medications.
- Determine the maximum quantity that may be dispensed
- Conduct on-line prospective drug utilization review
- Confirm the amount the pharmacy will be paid
- Submit the claim for payment
- Determine the patient's copayment

Your pharmacy's computer system takes care of many functions for you automatically. Pharmacy computer systems usually require that you complete each field before you go on to the next one. Therefore, it is the pharmacy's computer, rather than the PBM's that notifies you when a field is missing. Generally, if you enter the drug name, strength and quantity, the computer calculates the pricing information.

> **Note: Be careful to select the correct NDC number.** When you enter the drug name and strength, the pharmacy computer system may give you a choice of several different NDC numbers for generic equivalents and/or different package sizes. Check the original stock bottle to make sure that you select the correct NDC number. Using the wrong number can result in incorrect reimbursement or cause audit problems later. Some pharmacies avoid this problem by using bar code scanners to capture the correct NDC number directly off the manufacturer's stock bottle label.
>
> **Note:** The NDC number consists of 11 digits: the first five identify the manufacturer; the next four identify the name, strength and dosage form of the medication; the last two digits identify the package size. It is important that all 11 digits are correct. (See chapter entitled "Prescription Medication" for more information on NDC numbers.)

When the claim is submitted, the PBM will either accept the claim as submitted or send back a response indicating why the claim was not accepted.

Since many of these messages are triggered by data entry errors, you should check to make sure all data entered into the computer is accurate. Depending on the type of problem, you may need to check cardholder ID numbers, patient birth dates, NDC numbers, days supply, or other fields. Some rejection messages will require the pharmacist to get a prior authorization (PA) from the PBM or call the physician for changes to the prescription.

Processing third-party prescription clams may be one of your primary tasks when working in a pharmacy department. Remember that patients' plan numbers may change when insurance contracts are renewed, so be sure to give careful attention to your work and double-check all numbers you enter in the computer. Although following all third-party program procedures strictly is important to preventing claims rejections, it is also necessary in order to prevent problems when the pharmacy is audited by a PBM.

Third-Party Cost Controls

Formulary. To reduce ingredient costs, PBMs generally establish formularies — lists of medications that are covered (i.e., a positive formulary) or excluded from coverage (i.e., a negative formulary). These formularies commonly exclude certain classes of drugs such as: oral contraceptives, products used primarily for cosmetic purposes, weight control products, experimental medications, parenteral medications (other than insulin), and certain compounded medications. Formularies may only cover certain drugs within a therapeutic class and no others. Coverage restrictions can be complicated and often are not apparent until a claim is submitted to the PBM.

Figure 1

DAW Code Values
0 = No Product Selection Indicated
This is the field default value that is appropriately used for prescriptions where product selection is not an issue. Examples include prescriptions written for single source brand products and prescriptions written using the generic name and a generic product is dispensed.
1 = Substitution Not Allowed by Prescriber
This value is used when the prescriber indicates, in a manner specified by prevailing law, that the product is to be Dispensed As Written.
2 = Substitution Allowed – Patient Requested Product Dispensed
This value is used when the prescriber has indicated, in a manner specified by prevailing law, that generic substitution is permitted and the patient requests the brand product. This situation can occur when the prescriber writes the prescription using either the brand or generic name and the product is available from multiple sources.
3 = Substitution Allowed – Pharmacist Selected Product Dispensed
This value is used when the prescriber has indicated, in a manner specified by prevailing law, that generic substitution is permitted and the pharmacist determines that the brand product should be dispensed. This can occur when the prescriber writes the prescription using either the brand or generic name and the product is available for multiple sources.
4 = Substitution Allowed – Generic Drug Not in Stock
This value is used when the prescriber has indicated, in a manner specified by prevailing law, that generic substitution is permitted and the brand product is dispensed since a currently marketed generic is not stocked in the pharmacy. This situation exists due to the buying habits of the pharmacist, not because of the unavailability of the generic product in the market place.
5 = Substitution Allowed – Brand Drug Dispensed as a Generic
This value is used when the prescriber has indicated, in a manner specified by prevailing law, that generic substitution is permitted and the pharmacist is utilizing the brand product as the generic entity.
6 = Override
This value is used by various claims processors in very specific instances as defined by the claims processor and/or it's client(s).
7 = Substitution Not Allowed – Brand Drug Mandated by Law
This value is used when the prescriber has indicated, in a manner specified by prevailing law, that generic substitution is permitted but prevailing law or regulation prohibits the substitution of a brand product even though generic versions of the product may be available in the marketplace.
8 = Substitution Allowed – Generic Drug Not Available in Marketplace
This value is used when the prescriber has indicated, in a manner specified by prevailing law, that generic substitution is permitted and the brand product is dispensed since the generic is not currently manufactured, distributed, or is temporarily unavailable.
9 = Other
This value is reserved and currently not in use. NCPDP does not recommend use of this value at the present time. Please contact NCPDP if you intend to use this value and document how it will be utilized by your organization.

Source: National Council for Prescription Drug Programs, "NCPDP Data Element Dictionary"

Generic selection. Another way PBMs control prescription costs is by encouraging the use of generic medications. Payers often base reimbursement on generic prices when multiple-source medications are prescribed — whether or not brand-name medications are actually dispensed. PBMs may establish a "maximum allowable cost" (MAC) provision, originally used by the federal government for state Medicaid program reimbursement. A MAC is the maximum amount the payer will pay for a certain drug product. The federal list is referred to as the "federal upper limit" (FUL) list. Some state Medicaid programs have established their own "state MAC" lists that are more extensive than the federal guidelines. Many non-governmental plans have also adopted their own versions of MAC lists.

DAW. Sometimes physicians insist on a brand-name drug by indicating "dispense as written" or checking a "DAW box" on the prescription form. In every case, you must provide the proper "DAW code" when completing a claim. DAW code values are included in Figure 1. Be sure to use the proper code and know which codes are accepted by the various managed care plans — some plans do not use all of the codes. Always follow the established procedure in the pharmacy for reporting DAW codes. Some plans will not pay for multiple-source brand names even if the physician indicates DAW. Therefore, the patient must pay cash for all or part of the prescription at the time of pick-up. If in doubt, check with your pharmacist supervisor about how to bill these claims or how to charge these patients.

Therapeutic interchange. PBMs may encourage pharmacists to dispense a drug product that is therapeutically, but not generically equivalent to the product prescribed. Pharmacists may need to obtain authorization from the prescribing physician in order to make a therapeutic switch.

Quantity restrictions. PBMs often restrict the quantity of prescription medications that are covered. These restrictions prevent patients from getting unnecessarily large quantities of medications. A typical restriction is no more than one-month's supply (which is defined as 30 days in some plans and 34 days in others). Some plans that limit most prescriptions to a one-month supply will allow larger quantities for specified "maintenance medications" that are taken on a long-term basis for chronic conditions (e.g., high blood pressure medications). For example, if the patient is taking two tablets per day, a maximum of 100 tablets may be dispensed at one time, even though this is actually a 50-day supply. Another example would be allowing birth control tablets to be dispensed in up to a three-month supply.

Prior authorization. Most prior authorizations require physicians to call the insurance company. The insurance company will then authorize the prescription. Then the pharmacy may prepare and dispense the medication. Some plans specify that pharmacies must telephone the PBM to receive approval before they are allowed to dispense certain prescriptions. If the plan authorizes the prescription, you will be given a code that you can use to document the approval. You should follow your pharmacy's procedures for documenting the authorization. Authorization may be given for one transaction, several transactions, or a year's worth of transactions.

Drug utilization review. Most PBMs use drug utilization review (DUR) to monitor patterns of prescribing, dispensing and usage of prescription drugs. DUR may be prospective or retrospective. **Retrospective DUR** involves review of prescription claims databases well after the prescriptions have been dispensed. Since these programs are primarily educational, the focus is on alerting physicians and pharmacists to prescribing habits with the hope that they will be able to improve patients' outcomes using less costly medications.

Prospective DUR, on the other hand, occurs before the prescription is dispensed and results in alert messages being sent to the pharmacy's computer when problems are detected with the following:

- Duplication of therapy
- Allergies
- Dosage out of normal range
- Contraindications
- Drug interactions (categorized according to severity)
- Improper duration of therapy
- Unusual or unexpected patterns of prescription refills

When this occurs, the pharmacist must review the alert message and take appropriate action that may require a phone call to the physician, a discussion with the patient, or a call to the PBM to resolve the problem. These alerts may also result in a prescription being changed or not filled, if that is determined to be in the patient's best interests.

RECONCILIATION

When PBMs reimburse pharmacies for prescription claims, the check is usually accompanied by a "remittance advice" or "claims detail" or other document that shows the amount paid for each claim, the copayment amount and other messages that help explain how each claim is paid. This remittance advice is used to reconcile prescription claims with PBM payments.

> **Note: The claims reconciliation process is centralized in many large chain corporations. Although technicians working for these companies at the store level will not be checking the remittance advice itself, they may be asked to resolve problems. Nevertheless, knowing how the reconciliation process works will help technicians do better job during the claims adjudication process.**

Because of the difficulty in determining the accuracy of a payment response at the time of filling, a "back-end system" should be created that will allow the pharmacy to properly manage claims and collect the money that may be due from PBMs. A back-end system records the claim transaction, creates a receivable file, and then allows payments received to be matched against the claim. This helps to identify differences between expected payment and actual payments. A back-end claim management system will also help you determine:

- Was the adjudicated claim paid at all?

- Sometimes a claim does not make it onto a payment voucher. You need to check each claim against payment registers to be sure the claim was paid.

- Was the claim paid at the rate indicated by the adjudication response?

- The adjudicated response is what the PBM says it will pay. Payments may sometimes be adjusted by the PBM through its internal claim review process.

- If payment does not agree with the adjudicated response, you should check into this to find the reason. You may have to contact the PBM's help desk to determine the reason for the discrepancy.

- Was the claim paid at the correct contract rate?

- This is very difficult to determine unless you can determine which plan or network the patient is in. Some PBMs provide information on their remittance advice, which allows you to make that determination. In these cases you can compare your payment with your contracted rate.

- Was the claim paid in full?

- If the claim was paid in an amount other than the amount you anticipated, you should determine the payment differential and review why the claim payment varied from your anticipated payment.

- Payment variances can occur from MAC pricing, incorrect NDC number, incorrect quantity, or incorrect copayment.

CHARGEBACKS

Occasionally, a PBM may determine that it has paid a claim in error, or paid a claim incorrectly. They may bill back to the pharmacy the amount in question. Whenever receiving a chargeback, you should review the original claim, the adjudication response and the payment response to determine the facts involved in the charge-back request. If you have any issues with the chargeback, you should discuss the chargeback with the PBM. If you determine the chargeback is appropriate, you will need to make appropriate financial adjustments in accordance with your company's financial procedures. If you determine the chargeback is inappropriate, you should gather all appropriate documentation and call the PBM's help desk.

VERIFYING DELIVERY TO PATIENT

PBMs expect that patients receive every prescription for which it pays. You should be sure that you can document that every prescription that has been dispensed and billed—new or refill—has been received by either the patient or the patient's representative. This is an area that is often subject to audit. Some pharmacies may use signature logs, others may use a multi-part prescription form with a removable signature tag that contains all of the required prescription information and is affixed to a master log page that contains all the necessary legal language required by PBMs. Still others may have some type of electronic documentation of receipt. Some pharmacies use a delivery verification form that doubles as a HIPAA notification document.

Be sure to understand and follow the procedures in your pharmacy for documenting that the patient received the prescription. Without appropriate documentation, a payer could allege that the patient never received the prescription and attempt to recover payment for that prescription.

PARTIAL FILLS

If you find that there is not enough medication in stock to fill a prescription, your pharmacy may have to dispense a one-or two-day supply to hold the patient over until inventory can be replenished.

It is important that you do not bill the PBM twice for the prescription. Each pharmacy has its own procedures, so be sure to follow them carefully. It is a good idea to indicate on the prescription label the number of dosage units dispensed and the number owed. Also verify delivery, usually through a signature log or electronic system, at the time the patient picks up the remainder of the prescription.

CLAIM REVERSALS

Because some pharmacy systems generate a billing upon the completion of a prescription filling, there may be circumstances where a prescription that has been filled, billed and adjudicated needs to be reversed or "unbilled" when a patient does not receive the prescription—this is known as a **claim reversal.**

PBMs have developed procedures for pharmacies to follow when a claim that has been submitted and adjudicated must be reversed or "unbilled." This may occur if a prescription is filled and subsequently not picked up by the patient. Prescriptions may not be picked up by patients for a variety of reasons: the patient no longer needs the medication, the physician has changed the medication, the patient decided to get the prescription at another pharmacy, the patient forgot to pick it up, or the patient no longer wanted the prescription.

Each pharmacy should have appropriate procedures to address prescriptions that are not picked up. On a regular basis, you should review prescriptions that have not been picked up and determine with your pharmacist what procedures you should follow.

AUDITS

Although following all third-party program procedures strictly is important to preventing claim rejections, it is also necessary in order to prevent problems when the pharmacy is audited by a PBM. When a PBM performs an audit on a pharmacy, the auditor examines the pharmacy's records to make sure that there are prescriptions to cover all claims submitted to the PBM and that all of the information submitted on the claims was accurate. PBM auditors pay particular attention to making sure that a patient or their representative has signed for all prescriptions that have been billed to the PBM and that the DAW codes used on claims were accurate. If an auditor finds any discrepancies between the claims submitted to the PBM and the records in the pharmacy to back them up, the auditor may file a report that asks the pharmacy to make restitution, or pay money back to the PBM. If billing errors are numerous or large in magnitude, the pharmacy may be removed from the PBM's network of provider pharmacies. Thus, it is extremely important that as a pharmacy technician, you consider it your duty to submit claims that are accurate and adhere to all PBM guidelines in order to prevent such adverse consequences for your employer.

Acknowledgment: Some information in this chapter was adapted from:

Schafermeyer KW, *"Third-Party Prescription Program Evaluation,"* Chapter 10 in Effective Pharmacy Management, Eighth Edition (Alexandria, VA: National Community Pharmacists Association, 1996):317-354

Schafermeyer KW, *"The Impact of Managed Care on Pharmacy Practice,"* Chapter 19 in Navarro RP (ed.) Managed Care Pharmacy Practice (Gaithersburg, MD:Aspen Publications, 1999):451-473.

SELF-ASSESSMENT QUESTIONS CHAPTER IX

1. The upper limit of what a third-party program pays for multiple-source medications is known as a(n):
   a. AWP.
   b. DAW.
   c. HMO.
   d. MAC.

2. While you are entering prescription information into the computer a message appears stating that the prescribed medication is not covered and suggests another medication instead. It is apparent that the third-party program is using a(n):
   a. Capitation payment.
   b. Coinsurance.
   c. Formulary.
   d. Assignment of claims.

3. An organization that specializes in the management of the prescription drug program of a managed care organization is known as a:
   a. HMO.
   b. PA.
   c. PBM.
   d. POS.

4. A "dispense as written" provision:
   a. Allows pharmacies to be reimbursed for multiple-source brand-name drugs under some circumstances.
   b. Requires that pharmacies dispense the lowest cost generic equivalent.
   c. Is used primarily in indemnity or out-of-pocket payment.
   d. Requires a paper claim form for reimbursement.

5. When a managed care plan uses a tiered copayment
   a. Patients with greater income pay a larger portion of the prescription cost.
   b. Patients must pay more of their health care costs before their managed care plan pays for any prescription benefits.
   c. Patients pay 20 percent of the cost of higher-priced prescription drugs.
   d. Patients must pay more money when they receive a brand-name drug.

Answers:
1) d
2) c
3) c
4) a
5) d

PHARMACY TECHNICIAN COMPETENCY ASSESSMENT
CHAPTER IX

Description of Ability or Skill	Initials		Training Completed	
	Tech	R.Ph.	Date	Remarks
The technician trainee can differentiate among the various types of third-party prescription programs				
The technician trainee can locate and use information describing medication restrictions and exclusions required by major third-party plans.				
The technician trainee can describe the purpose of the various types of third-party program coverage limitations.				
The technician trainee can describe the three components of prescription reimbursement.				
The technician trainee can explain the purpose of patient cost sharing and differentiate among various types.				
The technician trainee can identify common data-entry errors that may cause a third-party claim to be rejected, and has developed a prevention check-list.				
The technician trainee can reconcile third-party claims.				
The technician trainee can use third-party signature logs.				

Chapter X
Non-Dispensing Duties

EDUCATIONAL OBJECTIVES

After studying the material in this chapter, the technician trainee should be able to:

- Describe how to place general orders for merchandise
- Understand the guidelines for ordering prescription medications from other pharmacy departments
- Identify outdated merchandise
- Understand the procedures for returning merchandise
- Stock and maintain pharmacy shelves
- Understand how to perform all needed cash register functions

INVENTORY CONTROL

The goal of any community pharmacy department is to stock enough merchandise to meet patient needs without having too much money tied up in inventory. It is a fine line; too many dollars invested in inventory results in an inefficient use of cash, while too few dollars will result in out-of-stocks, lost sales and unhappy patients. As the largest investment in the pharmacy, inventory must be managed properly. You will be responsible for helping pharmacists maintain the proper inventory level.

Purchasing

Buying from wholesalers. Most pharmacy departments place orders for prescription medications with their wholesaler (supplier) on a regular basis and receive the products the next day. Pharmacies generally buy most of their prescription medications from one major supplier and use a second wholesaler as a back-up supplier. Minimizing the number of orders improves efficiency because ordering stock and checking it in takes time and effort. Therefore, some pharmacies order two or three times a week, rather than daily.

> **Note:** Pharmacies that are part of a multiple-store corporation often maintain their own warehouse. If your pharmacy does this, the procedures used by your pharmacy may be different than the process explained in this chapter. A pharmacist will explain the procedure used by your pharmacy.

Buying from manufacturers. Most pharmacy departments use a secondary source for ordering medications as well; for example, buying medications directly from the manufacturer. The advantage of buying from a manufacturer is decreased costs. The disadvantages are that large quantities of products must be purchased at one time and orders may take several days or more to arrive.

Buying in large quantities. For example, a pharmacy department will typically sell much more of an antibiotic in the middle of the winter than in the middle of the summer. However, in the summer the manufacturer may offer a special low price on a large quantity, maybe enough for the entire winter. If accurate records from past years can identify the amount likely needed, a pharmacist or the company will be able to make an informed decision about whether and how much to order, provided funds are available.

> **Note:** Large size containers (500s and 1000s) usually have a lower per-unit cost than 100 count bottles; however, inventory investment and a slow rate-of-use often cancel out the advantage of the discount if the product is not dispensed frequently enough.

Generally, the stock size ordered is influenced by four factors:

1. How fast the product sells
2. How much time elapses between ordering and delivery
3. How much product must be purchased to get a good price
4. How important it is to avoid running out of stock, as with particular life-saving medications

Buying generics. Stocking generics is normally much less expensive than stocking brand-name medications. The more generics you dispense, the smaller the quantity of branded products you will have to carry in inventory, which lowers your inventory cost.

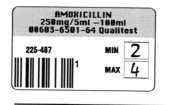

Sample shelf sticker

Reorder points and order-entry devices. You may wonder how you know when and how much to order. Some pharmacy departments have the reorder point and the reorder quantity printed or handwritten on a sticker attached to the edge of the stock shelf, usually under the product it describes. (See sample.) The reorder point identifies the minimum number of units to have on hand. When the stock quantity is at or below the reorder point number, this is the time to order more stock.

The reorder quantity is the maximum number of units to maintain in stock. In this example, if two units of amoxicillin 250 mg/5mL – 100 mL bottles remain on the shelf, you must order enough (two additional bottles) to have a total of four units in stock.

When reordering medication, your pharmacy department probably uses some type of an order entry device supplied by a wholesaler which is typically a rectangular unit that is a little larger than a hand-held calculator, like that shown on the right. Simply key the product's item number and order quantity into the device.

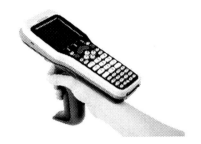

Example of an Order Entry Device

On some ordering devices, you do not need to key in any information. Instead, a scanning wand is used which operates by passing a light beam over the bar code of the NDC number or item number code. The bar code is the striped bars printed on the shelf label. You simply pass the wand over the code, then key-in the reorder quantity.

Once you have completed entering the order, put the order-entry device aside until the time when the order is normally transmitted to the wholesaler via telephone. In a few seconds, the order will be transmitted to the wholesaler's computer.

Ordering through the computer. Some pharmacies use what is known as a computerized "point of sale" (POS) system with which they can keep constantly-updated inventory records. The computer can be programmed with reorder points and the order quantities. As inventory is sold, the computer keeps track of stock and automatically reorders the appropriate quantity. When inventory falls to the reorder point, the computer adds that product to the list to be ordered.

At the end of the day, a pharmacist or technician will check the computer-generated list of items to be ordered. You may adjust the numbers to correct for seasonal changes or special circumstances (such as a flu epidemic). After the order is approved, the computer sends it to the wholesaler.

Ordering from another pharmacy department. If the pharmacy department where you work needs a medication in a hurry and has a good relationship among pharmacies in your area, these pharmacies may sell or transfer products to your pharmacy department in times of need. The cost of the goods is probably different than buying from your supplier unless the pharmacies order from the same sources. Your pharmacy will be responsible for picking up the medication, of course. Remember to note the addition to your inventory, if your pharmacy maintains a perpetual inventory for controlled substances.

Transferring controlled substances between pharmacies may be restricted in your state. In states where it is allowed, appropriate paperwork must be completed to document the transaction. (See chapter entitled, "Controlled Substances" for more information. If you have any questions, ask a pharmacist.)

Ordering patient requests. A patient may have been prescribed a medication which your pharmacy department does not normally stock. When this occurs, you will have to order it from the wholesaler and ask the patient to pick up the prescription the next day. Ask a pharmacist about your pharmacy's policy and procedure for special orders.

Receiving Goods

When an order is delivered to the pharmacy department, it should be checked in as soon as possible because unfilled prescriptions may be waiting for the medication to arrive. As a first step, verify that the number of cartons delivered matches the number shipped.

Along with the medication, you may receive self-adhesive product stickers. The number of individual stickers should match the number of units ordered and received. Applying the stickers to the product packages gives you a second check for counting the number of containers received. Leftover stickers or packages indicate an error.

Place a product sticker on each container so that it does not cover any important information such as the product name, bar code, lot number, expiration date, warnings, or directions for use. Some pharmacy departments have a designated spot where all product stickers should be placed on packages and bottles. All medication information should be visible so a pharmacist or pharmacy technician can confirm that the medication is the right medication and is not expired. Be sure to verify that stickers match products.

Once the order is checked in, record any shortages or omissions on the invoice and report them to a pharmacist. You may be asked to reorder items that were not shipped from the original supplier or to obtain them from another supplier. You should then sign and date the invoice. This indicates that the invoice is correct and can now be paid or should be paid only after the amount has been adjusted for the discrepancies in the order.

In some instances, the number of pieces and stickers will match each other but will not match the number of products ordered. When this happens, it usually signals that the wholesaler recognizes the shortages and has adjusted the billing accordingly. However, you should not assume this is the explanation; check it out to be sure.

Place the completed invoices in an area designated by a pharmacist. Controlled substances are invoiced separately and should be checked in, signed, and dated by a pharmacist.

Stocking Medications

As you restock the shelves (i.e., put incoming orders from supplier on the shelves), remember to rotate the stock (i.e., put new bottles at the back of the shelf and pull the older bottles forward). Always use the older bottles first before they expire. The expiration date is written on each package label. Check expiration dates on bottles as you handle them. Any expired medications should be brought to the attention of a pharmacist.

Another thing to do while restocking is to "face the stock bottles" (i.e., pull merchandise forward to the edge of the shelf).

You can learn much about medications while restocking. Become familiar with medication names, strengths, and dosage forms. You should also learn about medications that require special care, such as those that must be refrigerated or require compounding (mixing). Try to learn the medications on the speed shelf first because they can account for a significant percentage of all prescriptions dispensed in your pharmacy.

Checking for Expired Merchandise

According to the Food and Drug Administration, medications should not be sold to patients unless pharmacists, in their professional judgment, determine that the quantity dispensed will be used before the expiration date on the stock container. For example, if today is January 1, and you look at a container that has an expiration date of April 1 of this year, and the prescription calls for the patient to take one tablet a day, you can still dispense 60 tablets from that bottle since the last tablet would be used before the medication's expiration date. Expiration dates do not imply that a medication has full potency on the day before it expires and zero potency the day after. Medications gradually lose their strength over a period of time.

You must always be on the alert for expired or "short-dated" merchandise. Short-dated products are those which might expire before patients could use them. Check for short-dated merchandise when checking in orders. It only takes a second to look at the expiration date as you put product stickers on packages or put containers on the shelves. Your pharmacy department will have its own policy on what time frame constitutes short-dating.

From time to time, it may be necessary to check every bottle on the shelf for its expiration dating. This is usually done while dusting or cleaning the bays. Some pharmacy departments like to check for expired medications every three to six months. Doing so keeps inventory streamlined and minimizes the dollars invested in inventory unable to be sold.

Returning Merchandise

There are a variety of reasons and methods for returning expired or unwanted merchandise to the supplier. The supplier's response to the return depends on when the item was purchased and whether it has been opened. Also, suppliers differ on their return goods policies.

Merchandise ordered in error. Perhaps, for example, the person doing the ordering did not read the shelf sticker correctly and ordered 10 units instead of 01. In this situation, the merchandise can usually be returned by simply filling out a return sheet. The cost of having a wholesaler handle returns is high, so be accurate in your ordering.

Expired merchandise. Suppliers usually will take back expired merchandise if the package has not been opened. However, most will not take back "partials" (opened packages). Manufacturers sometimes will take back partially used containers of medication.

A wholesaler may choose not to take back expired merchandise, or the manufacturer of the product may insist that expired merchandise bypass the wholesaler and be returned directly to the manufacturer. When you return medication, you usually receive credit rather than cash. A pharmacy department may apply this credit toward an outstanding bill, or it may have the returned merchandise replaced by different products that are more frequently prescribed. In either case, you may be the one to complete the paperwork.

The procedure for returning expired products to the manufacturer varies from pharmacy to pharmacy. In general, expired products are sorted according to manufacturer. Obtain a "returned goods authorization form" from the manufacturer to expedite the returns.

Whether you return merchandise to the wholesaler, the warehouse, or the manufacturer, the procedure is basically the same. List the name, strength, dosage form and package size for each product, noting the exact quantity being returned and its cost. List partials as a fraction of the total. See the returned goods authorization form for detailed instructions. Box the merchandise and ship or mail it. Keep a copy of the list of returned goods and the mailing record or shipping receipt for your records.

As always, controlled substances require special handling and separate invoices. In any case, it is wise to take care of returns promptly for these reasons:
- Returns tie up money that may be needed for other purposes.
- Products to be returned take up storage space that could be put to better use.
- Some manufacturers will not take back expired products beyond a certain date after they expire.

Returning recalls. Occasionally the manufacturer will recall a medication from the marketplace due to production errors or other problems. The recall will describe the name, strength, dosage form, expiration date, and lot or batch number. You may be asked to help remove the product from the shelves, using the NDC number, expiration date, and lot number. You may also be asked to prepare the product for return and fill out the paperwork. Always keep a copy for your pharmacy department's records.

Maintaining Efficiency through Regular Routines

The pharmacy department's efficiency depends upon its being kept organized and well-stocked. As a pharmacy technician, some or all of that responsibility will be given to you. As you gain experience, you will know what has to be done and pharmacists will expect you to do it without being asked. Among your other duties, you will be expected to take care of the areas described in the following paragraphs.

Keep clean those areas visible to patients. The in-and out-windows must have clean counter surfaces and be free of clutter. (The in-or out-windows may, however, be appropriate places for patient education material.) If the prescription department has a waiting area, straighten the chairs and pamphlet racks, and stack the magazines throughout the day. The cleanliness of the pharmacy department reflects the professionalism and care of the pharmacists and the technicians working in it.

Keep supplies in good order and well-stocked. The pharmacy's efficiency depends on things being where they should be when they are needed. Since the pharmacy department consumes supplies all day long, you need to make sure that various size vials, bottles, and jars, prescription labels, prescription pads, auxiliary labels, and computer paper are always stocked in the pharmacy department.

Maintain stock. Your maintenance duties may include dusting and facing the OTC shelves; returning stock bottles to the prescription department shelves as soon as a pharmacist has checked and approved a prescription; calling in orders; verifying and shelving in-coming orders (remembering to rotate stock); checking expiration dates; and pulling expired bottles to be returned.

Check the bins of completed prescriptions. Examine the dates on the bags. If patients have not picked up prescriptions within several weeks, or within the time designated by your pharmacy department, call them to see if the prescriptions are still wanted. Your pharmacy department may have a specific procedure for handling prescriptions that may not be picked up.

SALES TRANSACTIONS

Using the Cash Register

If you have not already been taught how to use the cash register, ask to schedule some time for instruction. Because of the many kinds of registers in pharmacies across the country, instruction in the mechanics of ringing up a sale is not practical in this *Training Program*. Following are some transactions that require special attention.

Tax-exempt purchases. Prescription medications, baby formula, food supplements, and some home health-care items are not taxed in many states. Ask a pharmacist about the procedure for handling these sales in your state.

Senior-citizen discounts. Discounts are sometimes offered to people over 55 or 60. However, your pharmacy department's policy may exclude certain prescription medications. Also, the discount may have a maximum, for instance, $5.00 per purchase. Instead of offering a discount, some pharmacy departments offer coupons that can be redeemed for merchandise in the over-the-counter (OTC) area(s) of the pharmacy. Ask a pharmacist if your pharmacy department offers a senior-citizen discount. If so, find out the minimum eligibility age and how to apply the discount.

Personal charge accounts. In addition to payment by cash, check, or charge card, some pharmacy departments offer personal charge accounts for their prescription patients. Ask a pharmacist to explain the procedure for pharmacy department charge accounts, if appropriate.

Stocking and Organizing Transaction Supplies

If the cash register is placed where patients pick up their prescriptions, transaction supplies should be kept nearby:

- Small prescription bags and larger bags for holding several purchases.
- Stapler and staples
- Register slips, check-out, over-ring, and refund slips
- Blank charge card slips
- Pens and notepads
- Signature logs

Know the location and quantities of these supplies. You will probably be the person who keeps these items stocked and organized.

SELF-ASSESSMENT QUESTIONS CHAPTER X

1. Assume that the minimum order point for a product is four units and the maximum quantity is ten units. If there are six units in stock, how many should be ordered?
   a. 0
   b. 2
   c. 4
   d. 10

2. Assume that the minimum order point for a product is four units and the maximum is nine units. If there are two units in stock, how many should be ordered?
   a. 0
   b. 2
   c. 7
   d. 9

3. According to the *Training Program*, which of the following is NOT a factor that influences the size of a merchandise order?
   a. How fast the product sells
   b. How much time elapses between ordering and delivering
   c. How much product must be purchased to get a good price
   d. How much time is required to produce the product

4. If a product has an expiration date of April, 2008, it:
   a. May be dispensed until April 30, 2008.
   b. May be dispensed until April 1, 2008.
   c. Should be used by the patient by April 30, 2008.
   d. Should be used by the patient by April 1, 2008.

5. Which of the following best describes a distribution center commonly owned by multi-store corporations in which pharmacies may purchase medications from.
   a. Manufacturer
   b. Warehouse
   c. Wholesaler
   d. Drug company

Answers
1)   a
2)   c
3)   d
4)   c
5)   b

PHARMACY TECHNICIAN COMPETENCY ASSESSMENT
CHAPTER X

| Description of Ability or Skill | Initials | | Training Completed | |
	Tech	R.Ph.	Date	Remarks
The technician trainee can properly place a general order for merchandise.				
The technician trainee knows when and how to order prescription medication from other pharmacy departments.				
The technician trainee can successfully check for expired merchandise both when filling prescriptions and when receiving goods.				
The technician trainee knows when and how to return merchandise to suppliers.				
The technician trainee can stock and maintain pharmacy shelves efficiently.				
The technician trainee can successfully perform all needed functions at the cash register.				

Chapter XI
Drug and Medical Terminology
By: Brandon M. Williams

EDUCATIONAL OBJECTIVES

After studying the material in this chapter, the technician trainee should be able to:

- Identify word parts used in medical terminology
- Define common medical prefixes, word roots, and suffixes
- Use medical terminology to define the meaning of words used in pharmacy and other medical settings
- Use drug terminology to identify a drug product's therapeutic class and primary indications.

OVERVIEW

Knowledge of medical terminology is essential for any career in the medical field. While medical terminology appears foreign and confusing at first, developing a basic working vocabulary is not as difficult as it may seem. The key to developing this basic knowledge is understanding the meaning of the parts of the word; prefixes, suffixes, and word roots. A prefix is at the beginning of the word and usually indicates location, amount, or time. A word root is the basic meaning of the term. A suffix is at the end of the word and often indicates a condition or procedure. Combining vowels are used to connect suffixes to a root words and also make words easier to pronounce.

Examples of Medical Terminology

Prefix	Word root	C.V.*	Suffix	Word and definition
neuro- (nerve)	-		-pathy (disease)	**neuropathy-** any disease condition of the nervous system
-	hom (same)	eo	-stasis (steady)	**homeostasis-** the ability of the body to keep internal conditions stable
-	leuk (white)	o	-cyte (cell)	**leukocyte-** white blood cell
-	Erythr (red)	o	-cyte (cell)	**erythrocyte-** red blood cell
anti- (against)	pyret (fever)		-ic (pertaining to)	**antipyretic-** a class of drugs used to treat fever
hyper- (high)	glyc (sugar)		-emia (blood)	**hyperglycemia-** high concentration of sugar in the blood
hypo- (low)	-		-tension (pressure)	**hypotension-** low blood pressure

* CV = Combining vowel(s)

Even though medical terminology is very helpful to learn the meaning of words, there are instances where the word parts may mislead you in determining the true meaning of the word. For example, prognosis literally means "before knowledge." However, the actual definition is the forecast of the probable course of the disease.

The following are some additional prefixes, word roots, suffixes, and terms which are helpful for health professionals to know. In the following sections, there is also additional terminology associated with anatomy and physiology (see chapter entitled, Basic Anatomy & Disease States").

Prefixes   **Word Roots**

Prefix	Meaning
a-, an-	without, deficiency
ana-	excessive, again
anti-, ant-	against, opposing
auto-	self, same
cata-	down
epi-	On, upon
hemi-	one-half
idio-	one's own, self-produced
inter-	between
intra-	within
mal-	bad, a disorder
meta-	change or transformation
neo-	new or recent
onco-	tumor
pan-	all, entire
poly-	many
pro-	before
quadric-	four
sym, syn-	with, together

Word Root	Meaning
arthr/o	joint
arteri/o	artery
ather/o	fatty substance or plaque
carcin/o	cancer
card/I	heart
Cyst	bladder
cyt/o	cell
Derma	skin
Don't	teeth
gastr/o	stomach
hemat/o	blood
kinse/I	movement, motion
Lingu	tongue
lip/o	fat
my/o	muscle
nephr/o	kidney
ot/o	ear
pneum/o	lung
oste/o	bone

Suffixes

Suffix	Meaning
-algia	pain
-ectomy	surgical removal, excision
-esthesia	sensation
-genesis	formation, creation
-gram	a record of tracing
-graph	instrument
-graphy	process of recording
-ist	one who specializes in
-it is	inflammation
-meter	instrument used to measure
-ology	the study of
-oma	tumor
-osis	condition or process
-otomy	an temporary incision
-penia	deficiency
-phagia	eating
-plasty	surgical formation of
-rhage, -rhagia	excessive discharge

Common Medical Terms

Term	Definition
Acute	Short-term or rapid onset (opposite of chronic)
Anabolism	Building up body tissue from nutrients such as proteins; constructive metabolism
Analgesia	Loss of sensibility to pain
Anesthesia	Complete loss of sensation
Antiseptic	Preventing decay by killing or preventing the growth of microorganisms
Arthritis	Inflammation of one of more joints
Benign	Not harmful or life-threatening and does not spread (opposite of malignant)
Carcinoma	A cancerous, malignant or life-threatening tumor
Cardiac	Pertaining to the heart
Catabolism	Creating energy from breaking down fats or carbohydrates; destructive metabolism
Cancer	Disorder in which the body produces an excessive amount of dysfunctional cells that may multiply and invade nearby cells and organs possibly impairing their function and decreasing the body's ability to produce functional cells
Chronic	Long-term or constant (opposite of acute)
Edema	Excessive amount of fluid in a tissue
Glucosuria	Abnormal presence of glucose in the urine
Hemiplegia	Paralysis of one side of the body
Hyperesthesia	Excessive sensibility to stimuli
Hypernatremia	Excessive amount of sodium in the blood
Hyponatremia	Deficient amount of sodium in the blood
Hypervolumia	Excessive amount of fluid in a body tissue; also called edema
Hypovolemia	Deficient amount of fluid in a body tissue; also called dehydration
Idiopathic	Denoting a disease of an unknown cause
Lipid	Fat
Malignant	Harmful, life-threatening and tends to spread
Metastasis	Transfer of disease from one organ to another as seen in cancer
Metabolism	The sum of chemical reactions that provide energy for vital processes in the body
Oncogenic	Causing tumor formation
Oncology	The study concerning the diagnosis, treatment and prevention of tumors
Parenteral	Injection or introduction into body via any route other than by mouth
Pediatrics	Branch of medicine concerned with the development and diseases of children
Podiatry	Branch of medicine concerned with diseases and injuries of the foot
Polydipsia	Excessive thirst; often seen in patients with diabetes
Polyphagia	Excessive eating; often seen in patients with diabetes
Polyuria	Excessive urination; often seen in patients with diabetes
Prognosis	Forecast of the probable course of a disease
Prophylaxis	Prevention of disease; preventative treatment
Quadriplegia	Paralysis of all four limbs
Sclerosis	A hardening especially from inflammation
Sepsis	Presence of pathogenic organisms or toxins
Sign	Evidence of a disease state such as a fever
Spasm	Involuntary muscle contraction, convulsion
Symptom	An effect observed by the patient (e.g., pain)
Syndrome	Aggregate signs and symptoms of a disease

DRUG TERMINOLOGY

Many times the class of a drug and what condition the drug may treat can be determined by looking at the generic name of a drug. The following table lists examples with the generic drug name followed by the brand name in parenthesis.

Condition treated	Generic drug name prefix/root/suffix	Drug class	Generic (brand) drug name examples
Allergies	-atadine	Antihistamine	Desloratadine (Clarinex) Loratadine (Claritin) Olopatadine (Patanol)
	-izine	Antihistamine	Cetirizine (Zyrtec)
Alzheimer's/ demetia	-pezil	Acetylcholinesterase inhibitor	Donepezil (Aricept)
Anxiety/ Sedative	-bital	Barbiturate	Amobarbital (Amytal) Butabarbital (Butisol) Pentobarbital Phenobarbital Secobarbital (Seconal)
	-toin	Anticonvulsant	Albutoin (Peganone) Fosphenytoin (Cerebyx) Phenytoin (Dilantin)
	-zepam	Benzodiazepine	Clonazepam (Klonopin) Diazepam (Valium) Flurazepam Lorazepam (Ativan) Oxazepam (Serax) Quazepam (Doral) Temazepam (Restoril)
	-zolam	Benzodiazepine	Alprazolam (Xanax) Estazolam Midazolam (Versed) Triazolam (Halcion)
Arthritis	-icam	NSAID	Meloxicam (Mobic) Piroxicam (Feldene)
Asthma	-lukast	Leukotriene receptor antagonist	Montelukast (Singulair) Zafirlukast (Accolate)
	-terol	Beta2-agonist	Albuterol (Proventil) Arformoterol (Brovana) Bitolterol (Tornalate) Formoterol (Perforomist) Levalbuterol (Xopenex) Pirbuterol (Maxair) Salmeterol (Serevent)

Condition treated	Generic drug name prefix/root/suffix	Drug class	Generic (brand) drug name examples
Bacterial infection	Cef-	Antibiotic (cephalosporin)	Cefaclor (Raniclor) Cefadroxil Cefazolin Cefdinir (Omnicef) Cefditoren (Spectracef) Cefixime (Suprax) Cefotaxime (Claforan) Cefotetan (Cefotan) Cefprozil (Cefzil) Ceftriaxone (Rocephin) Cefuroxime (Ceftin)
	-cillin	Antibiotic (penicillin)	Amoxicillin (Amoxil, Trimox) Ampicillin (Prencipen) Dicloxacillin Nafcillin Oxacillin Piperacillin Ticarcillin (Ticar)
	-floxacin	Antibiotic (quinolone)	Ciprofloxacin (Cipro) Gemifloxacin (Factive) Levofloxacin (Levaquin) Lomefloxacin (Maxaquin) Moxifloxacin (Avelox) Norfloxacin (Noroxin) Ofloxacin (Floxin)
	-mycin	Antibiotic (nonspecific)	Azithromycin (Zithromax) Clarithromycin (Biaxin) Clindamycin (Cleocin) Daptomycin (Cubicin) Erythromycin (EryTabs) Kanamycin (Kantrex) Lincomycin (Lincocin) Neomycin (Neosporin) Streptomycin Tobramycin (Tobradex) Vancomycin (Vancocin)
	-prim	Antibiotic (trimethoprim)	Trimethoprim (Bactrim)
	-pristin	Antibiotic (streptogramin)	Dalfopristin and Quinupristin (Synercid)
Benign Prostate Hyperplasia (BPH)	-zosin	Alpha blocker	Doxazosin (Cardura) Prazosin (Minipress) Terazosin (Hytrin)

Condition treated	Generic drug name prefix/root/suffix	Drug class	Generic (brand) drug name examples
Blood clot prevention	-grel	Antiplatelet agent	Clopidogrel (Plavix)
Depression	-italopram	Selective serotonin receptor inhibitor	Citalopram (Celexa) Escitalopram (Lexapro)
	-oxetine	Selective serotonin receptor inhibitor	Duloxetine (Cymbalta) Fluoxetine (Prozac, Sarafem) Paroxetine (Paxil)
	-pramine	Tricyclic antidepressant	Clomipramine (Anafranil) Desipramine (Norpramin) Imipramine (Tofranil) Trimipramine (Surmontil)
	-triptyline	Tricyclic antidepressant	Amitryptyline Nortryptyline (Pamelor) Protryptyline (Vivactal)
Diabetes	-formin	Biguanide	Metformin (Glucophage)
	-glitazone	Thiazolidinedione	Pioglitazone (Actos) Rosiglitazone (Avandia)
Erectile dysfunction	-afil	Phosphodiesterase-5 inhibitor	Sildenafil (Viagra) Tadafil (Cialis) Vardenafil (Levitra)
Fungal infection	-conazole	Miconazole derivatives	Fluconazole (Diflucan) Econzole (Spectazole) Itraconazole (Sporanox) Ketoconazole Miconazole (Micatin) Oxiconazole (Oxistat) Sertaconzole(Ertaczo) Sulconazole(Exelderm) Voriconazole (Vfend)
GERD/ Heartburn	-tidine	H2-antagonist	Cimetidine (Tagamet) Famotidine (Pepcid) Nizatidine (Axid) Ranitidine (Zantac)
	-prazole	Proton pump inhibitor (PPI)	Esomeprazole (Nexium) Lansoprazole (Prevacid) Omeprazole (Prilosec) Pantoprazole (Protonix) Rabeprazole (Aciphex)

Condition treated	Generic drug name prefix/root/suffix	Drug class	Generic (brand) drug name examples
Hyperlipidemia (high cholesterol) and/or Hypertriglyceridemia (high triglycerides)	-statin or -vastatin	HMG-CoA reductase inhibitor	Atorvastatin (Lipitor) Fluvastatin (Lescol) Lovastatin (Mevacor) Pravastatin (Pravachol) Rosuvastatin (Crestor)
	-imibe	2-azetidinone	Ezetimibe (Zetia)
	-fibrate	Fibric acid derivative	Fenofibrate (Tricor, Triglide)
Hypertension (High blood pressure)	-dipine	Calcium channel blocker (CCB)	Amlodipine (Norvasc) Felodipine (Plendil) Isradipine (DynaCirc) Nifedipine (Adalat, Procardia) Nicardipine (Cardene) Nisoldipine (Sular)
	-olol	Beta blocker	Acebutolol (Sectral) Atenolol (Tenormin) Bisoprolol (Zebeta) Esmolol (Brevibloc) Metoprolol tartrate (Lopressor) Metoprolol succinate (Toprol) Propranolol (Inderal) Timolol (Blocadren)
	-pril	ACE inhibitor (ACE-I)	Benazepril (Lotensin) Captopril (Capoten) Enalapril (Vasotec) Fosinopril (Monopril) Lisinopril (Prinivil, Zestril) Quinapril (Accupril) Ramipril (Altace) Trandolapril (Mavik)
	-sartan	Angiotensin receptor blocker (ARB)	Candesartan (Atacand) Irbesartan (Avapro) Losartan (Cozaar, Hyzaar) Olmesartan (Benicar) Telmisartan (Micardis) Valsartan (Diovan)
	-semide	Loop diuretic	Furosemide (Lasix) Torsemide (Demadex)
	-thiazide	Thiazide diuretic	Chlorothiazide (Diuril) Hydrochlorothiazide Methyclothiazide (Enduron)

Condition treated	Generic drug name prefix/root/suffix	Drug class	Generic (brand) drug name examples
Hypertension (High blood pressure) (continued)	-zolamide	Carbonic anhydrase inhibitor	Acetazolamide Methazolamide
	-zosin	Alpha blocker	Doxazosin (Cardura) Prazosin (Minipress) Terazosin (Hytrin)
Migraine	-triptan	Serotonin 5-HT agonist	Almotriptan (Axert) Eletriptan (Relpax) Frovatriptan (Frova) Naratriptan (Amerge) Rizatriptan (Maxalt) Sumatriptan (Imitrex) Zolmitriptan (Zomig)
Nausea and vomiting	-setron	Serotonin 5-HT$_3$ antagonists	Alosetron (Lotronex) Dolasetron (Anzemet) Granisetron (Kytril) Ondansetron (Zofran) Palonosetron (Aloxi)
Osteoporosis	-dronate	Biphosphonate	Alendronate (Fosamax) Ibandronate (Boniva) Risendronate (Actonel)
Pain	-adol	Nonnarcotic analgesic	Tramadol (Ultram)
	-codone	Opiates/ narcotic analgesics	Hydrocodone (Lortab, Vicodin, Lorcet, Oxycodone (Oxycontin, Percocet)
	-coxib	COX-2 inhibitor	Celecoxib (Celebrex)
	-eridine	Pethidine derivative	Meperidine (Demerol)
	-morphone	Opiates/ narcotic analgesics	Hydromorphone (Dilaudid) Oxymorphone (Opana)
	-profen	NSAID	Fenoprofen (Nalfon) Flurbiprofen (Ansaid) Ibuprofen (Advil, Midol, Motrin) Ketoprofen
Psychosis	-peridone	Antipsychotic (atypical)	Paliperidone (Invega) Risperidone (Risperdal)
	-apine	Antipsychotic (atypical)	Clozapine (Clozaril) Loxapine (Loxitane) Olanzapine (Zyprexa) Quetiapine (Seroquel)

Condition treated	Generic drug name prefix/root/suffix	Drug class	Generic (brand) drug name examples
Viral infection	-amivir	Neuraminidase inhibitors	Oseltamivir (Tamiflu) Zanamivir (Relenza)
	-mantadine	Viral uncoating inhibitors	Amantadine (Symmetrel) Rimantadine (Flumadine)
	-navir	Protease inhibitor	Atazanavir (Reyataz) Darunavir (Prezista) Fosamprenavir (Lexiva) Indinavir (Crixivan) Nelfinavir (Viracept) Ritonavir (Norvir) Saquinavir (Invirase) Tipranavir (Aptivus)
	vir or any name containing "vir"	Antiviral (nonspecific)	Abacavir (Epzicom) Acyclovir (Zovirax) Cidofovir (Vistide) Famciclovir (Famvir) Nevirapine (Viramune) Penciclovir (Denavir) Tenofovir (Viread) Valacyclovir (Valtrex)
	-vudine	Nuceloside reverse transcriptase inhibitor	Lamivudine (Combivir) Stavudine (Zerit) Zidovudine (Retrovir)

As with medical terminology, there are instances in drug terminology where the parts of the word may mislead you. For example, the generic name of Abilify is aripiprazole. Therefore, using the table above, one would expect that Abilify would be used for GERD or heartburn. However, Abilify is actually an antipsychotic used for the treatment of bipolar mania and schizophrenia. Many times, a medication may also be used to treat several conditions other than the one listed in the table above. For example, some beta blockers used to treat high blood pressure may also be used to treat heart failure. Therefore, even though drug terminology can be very useful, there are exceptions that may mislead you at times.

SELF-ASSESSMENT QUESTIONS CHAPTER XI

1. Which of the following best describes an *antihypertensive*?
   a. A drug used to treat high blood pressure
   b. A drug used to treat fever, pain, and headaches
   c. A drug used to treat high cholesterol
   d. A drug used to treat seizures

2. *Hyperlipidemia* is best characterized by which of the following?
   a. An excess amount of fats in the blood
   b. A deficiency of the amount of fats in the blood
   c. A metabolic disorder characterized by symptoms of glucose intolerance
   d. A higher than normal blood pressure

3. Which of the following best describes *neurology*?
   a. The branch of medicine concerned with diseases and injuries of the foot.
   b. The branch of medicine concerned with the development and diseases of children.
   c. The study concerning the diagnosis, treatment and prevention of tumors.
   d. The study of the nervous system and its disorders or diseases.

4. Which of the following is the best definition of *prophylaxis*?
   a. The prevention of disease or a preventative treatment
   b. A state of well-being
   c. A condition characterized by severe diarrhea
   d. A condition characterized by the heart failing to pump blood

5. Which of the following best describes *oncology*?
   a. The branch of medicine concerned with diseases and injuries of the foot.
   b. The branch of medicine concerned with the development and diseases of children.
   c. The study concerning the diagnosis, treatment and prevention of tumors.
   d. The study of the nervous system and its disorders or diseases.

Answers:
1) a
2) a
3) d
4) a
5) c

PHARMACY TECHNICIAN COMPETENCY ASSESSMENT

CHAPTER XI

	Initials		Training Completed	
Description of Ability or Skill	**Tech**	**R.Ph.**	**Date**	**Remarks**
The technician trainee can properly identify word parts in medical terms.				
The technician trainee properly uses medical terminology.				
The technician trainee spells common medical terms correctly.				
The technician trainee asks the pharmacist how to pronounce unfamiliar terms.				

Sources:

Enrlich, Ann, Medical Terminology for Health Professionals, Fouth Edition, (Albany, NY: Delmar Learning, 2001)

United States Adopted Names (USAN) Stem List. USAN Council. Approved Jan 26, 2007. Updated Jan 2008. Accessed Feb11, 2008. http://198.178.213.111/ama1/pub/upload/mm/365/stem_list-1-08.pdf

The use of stems in the selection of International Nonproprietary Names (INN) for pharmaceutical substances. © World Health Organization 2006. Accessed Feb 11, 2008. http://www.who.int/medicines/services/inn/RevisedFinalStemBook2006.pdf

Chapter XII
Basic Anatomy and Disease States
By: Brandon M. Williams

EDUCATIONAL OBJECTIVES

After studying the material in this chapter, the technician trainee should be able to:

- List the organ systems in the body
- Recognize anatomical structures
- Describe the general functions of the body's organ systems
- Use basic medical terminology associated with basic human anatomy and physiology
- Identify medical conditions consistent with each organ system

---

OVERVIEW

Understanding how medications work requires knowledge of anatomy and physiology. These complimentary branches of science provide the critical concepts of the relationship between structure and function of the body. Anatomy is the art of exploring the structure and position of body parts and their relationships to one another. Physiology is the study of the function of those body parts. Body parts that are made up of two or more tissues and carry out specific functions are called organs.

"Homeostasis" is the body's ability to maintain relatively stable internal conditions even when subjected to fluctuating environmental conditions. The body's organ systems act to preserve homeostasis so that the body operates properly. Learning about body structure and function presents a good opportunity to practice the medical terminology associated with the body's organ systems and become familiar with common medical conditions and treatments, including the proper use of medications.

ORGAN SYSTEMS

The Skeletal and Muscular Systems

The skeletal and muscular systems provide support and protection for the body's organs, allow for shape and movement, warmth, and posture. The skeleton is made up of bones, cartilage, ligaments, and joints.

There are 206 bones in the body which make up the majority of the skeletal system. Cartilages occur only in isolated areas, such as the nose, parts of the ribs and the joints. Ligaments connect bone and reinforce joints, allowing required movements while restricting motions in other directions. Joints, the junctions between bones, provide for the remarkable mobility of the skeleton without impairing its immense strength.

Our bodies contain skeletal, smooth and cardiac muscles. There are more than 600 skeletal muscles, which enable the body to perform a wide variety of activities. Skeletal muscles, also known as voluntary muscles, are attached to bones by tendons. Smooth muscle is muscle that is not under conscious control (involuntary) such as the muscles involved in digestion. Other smooth muscles, such as those involved in breathing, can be controlled to some extent but still work without conscious effort. Cardiac muscle is a special type of involuntary muscle found in heart tissues that allows the heart to pump continuously without conscious control.

Common Terminology Associated with the Skeletal and Muscular Systems
- **Arthr/o** – Joint.
- **Cartilage** - A specialized tissue that protects the ends of the bones by creating a smooth surface facilitating motion.
- **Chondr/o** - Cartilage.
- **Costa, costal** - Ribs.
- **Ligaments** - Connective tissue that connects one bone to another bone.
- **My/o** - Muscle.
- **Ossi - , oste/o** - Bone.
- **Sarc/o** - Flesh, muscle.
- **Spasm, spasm/o, spasm** - Involuntary muscle contraction; convulsion; cramp.
- **Tendon** - A tissue that connects muscles to bone.

Common Conditions and Diseases of the Skeletal and Muscular Systems
- **Arthritis** - An inflammation of one or more joints, which can be accompanied by pain, swelling or loss of function.
- **Gout** - A condition created by a buildup of uric acid in joints and tendons that promotes an inflammatory reaction resulting in sudden and excruciating pain. Most commonly involved are the feet, especially the big toe. Elevated levels of uric acid may complicate into kidney stones if left untreated.
- **Myalgia** - Muscle pain or tenderness.
- **Myosclerosis** - Abnormal hardening of muscle tissue.

- **Ostealgia** - Any pain in the bone resulting from a bone abnormality.
- **Osteoarthritis** - A degenerative disease of the joints in which cartilage that acts as a cushion between bones is worn away resulting in joint inflammation caused by the repeated bone-to-bone contact. Severity usually increases with age.
- **Osteoporosis** - A thinning of the bone making the bone more brittle and more susceptible to fracture; usually associated with a lack of calcium.
- **Rheumatoid arthritis** – An autoimmune disorder in which cartilage is destroyed resulting in joint inflammation, pain, weakness, fatigue, and stiffness. Rheumatoid arthritis can strike patients at any age. Some viral infections can cause temporary rheumatoid symptoms.
- **Sprain** - Injury to a joint (such as the knee, wrist, or ankle) usually caused by the overuse or overstrain of the joint resulting in stretching of the ligaments.
- **Strain** - Injury to a muscle, tendon or ligament resulting overextension or overstretching.
- **Tendonitis** - Inflammation of a tendon.

The Cardiovascular System

The cardiovascular system distributes oxygen throughout the body and helps remove carbon dioxide and waste products.

The heart is the pump that propels blood through the cardiovascular system. It is a muscle about the size of a fist and is divided into four chambers. The two atria, at the top, allow the return of blood from circulation and the two ventricles, at the bottom, force blood out of the heart. As blood flows into the atria, valves within the heart open and close in response to pressure changes, permitting passage of blood into the ventricles. The ventricles contract to drive the blood out of the heart, and then relax to allow more blood to flow in.

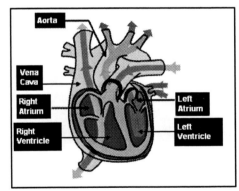

Blood pressure is characterized by the contraction and relaxation of the ventricles. When the ventricles contract, this is the systolic phase and when they relax, this is the diastolic phase. Blood pressure is read as the systolic pressure over the diastolic pressure (e.g., 120/80 mm Hg). Heart rate (HR), or pulse, is measured in beats per minute (BPM) (e.g., 60 BPM).

Blood is composed of two elements which are plasma and formed elements. Plasma consists of mostly water and some proteins, which are involved in blood clotting. The formed elements consist of red blood cells, white blood cells and platelets. Red blood cells transport oxygen to tissues and take carbon dioxide away from tissues; white blood cells aid in immunity; and platelets aid in the clotting of the blood.

Common Terminology Associated with the Cardiovascular System

- **Angioplasty** - The surgical repair of a blood vessel.
- **Artery** - Blood vessels that transports oxygenated blood away from the heart to body cells and tissues.
- **Capillaries** - Very small blood vessels where oxygen from the red blood cells is exchanged for carbon dioxide.
- **Cardi/o** - Heart.
- **Cardiology** - The study of the structure, functions, and disorders of the heart.
- **Cholesterol** - A type of lipid (i.e., fat) that circulates in the blood and can form plaques that can block blood vessels.
- **Electrocardiogram (ECG)** - A graphic representation of heart contractions made by an electrocardiograph, which can be used to diagnosis certain heart problems.
- **Erythrocyte** - Red blood cell that transports oxygen to body tissues and organs.
- **Hem/o, hemat/o** - Blood.
- **Hemoglobin** – An iron-containing protein found in red blood cells that carries oxygen from the lungs to body organs and tissues, and carries carbon dioxide from the body organs and tissues to the lungs for exhalation.
- **High-density lipoprotein (HDL)** - Also known as "good cholesterol," which transports unneeded cholesterol back to the liver and does not contribute to plaque on artery walls.
- **Low-density lipoprotein (LDL)** - Also known as "bad cholesterol," which can accumulate as plaque and block blood vessels
- **Myocardial** - Muscle of the heart
- **Plaque** - An accumulation of cholesterol in a blood vessel often resulting in a restricted blood flow and insufficient oxygen being transported to the tissues.

Common Conditions and Diseases of the Cardiovascular System

- **Anemia** - A reduction in the number of red blood cells and hemoglobin resulting in the decreased ability of red blood cells to transport oxygen to body cells and tissues .
- **Angina** – Chest pain that may radiate to the arms, jaw, neck, abdomen, or back but not as severe as a heart attack. Angina may be caused by exercise or a decrease in the blood supply to the heart.
- **Arrhythmia** – Irregular heartbeat often caused by hypertension, ischemic heart disease (IHD), or certain medications.
- **Arteriosclerosis** - A condition in which artery walls become thick and stiff usually because of increasing age.
- **Bradycardia** - (Slow heart rate) HR < 60 BPM.
- **Congestive Heart Failure (CHF)** - Condition in which the heart fails to pump blood efficiently, resulting in severe complications such as arrhythmias and death.
- **Embolism** - An object, such as a blood clot, which dislodges and travels through the bloodstream until it blocks a smaller blood vessel, thereby cutting off blood flow. Blood clots in veins often travel to the lungs where they can block blood flow from the heart to the lungs, preventing or reducing blood oxygenation.
- **Endocarditis** - Inflammation of the endocardium, the inner layer of the heart; often caused by a bacterial infection. The heart valves are often involved with some impairment in their function. Long courses of antibiotics are often used for treatment.

- **Hemorrhage** - Bleeding or a flow of blood due to trauma or a wound.
- **Hypertension** - High blood pressure characterized by an increase in blood pressure during heart contraction (systolic blood pressure) or relaxation (diastolic blood pressure). Hypertension is diagnosed as a systolic blood pressure of 140 or greater or a diastolic blood pressure of 90 or greater.
- **Ischemic Heart Disease (IHD)** – Obstruction of the blood supplied to the heart due to a buildup of lipids or fat in the arteries.
- **Leukemia** - Cancer in the bone marrow which prevents the formation of functional or mature white and red blood cells leading to deficient immunity, anemia, and increased susceptibility to infection.
- **Myocardial infarction** - Damage to the heart muscle resulting from blocked coronary arteries, which prevents sufficient oxygen being supplied to the heart; also known as a "heart attack."
- **Stroke** - A serious neurological condition caused by a decrease of oxygen supplied to the brain that can result in weakness, loss of control over muscles, difficulty speaking, and/or death. Strokes may be caused by either a blockage of a blood vessel in the brain or from a hemorrhage from a damaged blood vessel in the brain.
- **Tachycardia** - Rapid heart rate. (HR > 100 BPM).
- **Thrombus** - A clot that forms in a blood vessel and blocks blood flow.

The Respiratory System

The primary function of the respiratory system is ventilation. Ventilation is the process of moving air into and out of the body through inhalation and exhalation. Upon exhalation, the respiratory system eliminates carbon dioxide from the blood stream; upon inhalation the blood absorbs oxygen from the lungs. This exchange of carbon dioxide for oxygen takes place by diffusion at the respiratory membrane, also called the air-blood barrier, which is much thinner than a sheet of tissue paper. The blood transports oxygen from the lungs to cells, organs, and tissues, and carries carbon dioxide from the body back to the lungs to be expelled.

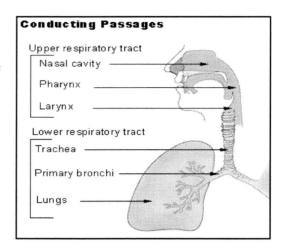

The lungs expand and collapse with aid from the diaphragm, which contracts during inhalation to bring air into the lungs and relaxes during exhalation to move air out of the lungs.

As air is inhaled through the nose, it is filtered, warmed, and moistened. It then moves into the pharynx, also known as the throat, which houses the tonsils, exposing the immune system to inhaled organisms. Next, the air passes through the larynx where the vocal cords are located and then travels through the trachea, or windpipe, which divides into two primary bronchial tubes, leading to the lungs. Inside the lungs, the bronchial tubes branch out into smaller and smaller bronchi, collectively called the respiratory tree.

Common Terminology Associated with the Respiratory System

- **Apnea** - An absence of spontaneous respiration.
- **Asphyxia** - Abnormal or pathologic changes caused by an absence of oxygen.
- **Aspiration** – The act of inhaling a foreign substance into the lungs, often after vomiting.
- **Dyspnea** - Shortness of breath.
- **Expiration** - The act of breathing out as the diaphragm relaxes.
- **Hyperventilation** - A condition characterized by rapid breathing resulting in decreased carbon dioxide levels and increased oxygen levels producing faintness, tingling of the fingers and toes, and possibly loss of consciousness.
- **Inhalation** - The act of breathing in as the diaphragm contracts.
- **Respiratory rate** - Also known as breaths per minute which is an important numeric value used for diagnosing respiratory conditions. The normal numeric value range is 15 to 20 breaths per minute.
- **Rhinorrhea** - An excessive flow of mucus from the nose (runny nose).

Common Conditions and Diseases of the Respiratory System

- **Allergic rhinitis** - Nasal inflammation characterized by an increased flow of mucus; caused by allergies.
- **Asthma** - A breathing disorder, often triggered by allergies or exercise, resulting in constriction of the bronchi. Asthma is often accompanied by tightness in the chest, coughing, wheezing and difficulty in breathing. Asthmatic episodes can range from mild coughing and wheezing to life-threatening breathing problems.
- **Chronic bronchitis** - Inflammation of the bronchi; usually caused by an infection in which the patient has a productive cough and difficulty getting sufficient oxygen. Some patients may have a bluish tint to lips or skin.
- **Chronic Obstructive Pulmonary Disease (COPD)** - A condition characterized by emphysema and chronic bronchitis usually caused by smoking; resulting in difficulty in breathing and increased risk of infection.
- **Cystic fibrosis** - Genetic disorder affecting mostly Caucasian populations where excessive amounts of thick mucus blocks the airways, resulting in wheezing, cough, and increased susceptibility to bacterial infections.
- **Emphysema** - A condition characterized by shortness of breath; usually caused by smoking. Some patients may have a pinkish tint to the face and may gasp for air.
- **Influenza** - An acute, highly contagious viral respiratory infection (also known as the flu), which is spread by coughing, sneezing and sharing items such as food utensils.
- **Laryngitis** - Inflammation of the larynx (voice box) resulting in temporary inability to speak normally.
- **Lung Cancer** – Disorder in which non-functional cells or tumors are produced in the lungs, causing pain, coughing, impairment of lung function. Lung cancer is often caused by smoking and often spreads to other organs.
- **Pertussis** - A contagious bacterial infection resulting in a loud, deep coughing; also known as whooping cough.
- **Pharyngitis** - Inflammation of the pharynx or throat.
- **Pneumonia** - Disease of the lungs characterized by inflammation of the lungs and congestion; often caused by bacteria or viruses.
- **Sinusitis** - Infection and inflammation of the membranes lining the sinuses.
- **Tonsillitis** - Infection and inflammation of the tonsils.

The Lymphatic and Immune Systems

The lymphatic and immune systems work together to protect us from bacterial and viral infections. Without the network of lymphatic vessels and tissues scattered throughout our bodies, the immune system would be desperately impaired. It filters out organisms that could harm us and produces specialized white blood cells (called lymphocytes) and antibodies. The largest lymphoid organ is the spleen, but the thymus, lymph nodes and tonsils are also part of the lymphatic system.

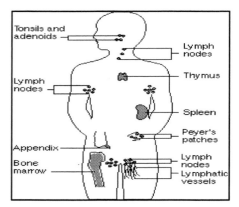

The spleen, located on the left side of the abdomen, cleans the blood of defective blood cells; removes debris, bacteria, viruses, and toxins; and stores certain white blood cells known as lymphocytes. Lymphocytes are the major warriors of the immune system protecting the body against foreign invaders. Some of these specialized white blood cells can also travel to the thymus to mature and wait to be called upon by the immune system.

Lymph (a creamy fluid containing lymphocytes, proteins, and fats) passes through the lymph nodes where microorganisms are destroyed. The tonsils (and adenoids), located in the throat, collect and remove pathogens that enter the body via inhaled air or ingested food.

Common Terminology of the Lymphatic and Immune Systems

- **Allergen** - Any substance capable of causing or inducing an allergic response.
- **Allergy** - An altered reaction of body tissues in response to an allergen that affects some people who are sensitive to that allergen but not others.
- **Antigen** - A substance such as a bacteria or a virus that the body recognizes as foreign.
- **Antibody** - A protein produced by the immune system that targets a specific antigen to inhibit it from invading the body cells and tissues.
- **Antibiotic** - A medication that is used to stop growth of bacteria but is not effective in viral infections.
- **Antiviral** - A medication used to treat viral infections or provide temporary immunity.
- **Antihistamine** - A medication that blocks histamine, a type of allergen that is produced by white blood cells, to control allergic reactions.
- **Bacteria** - Name given to a group of single-celled microorganisms. Some bacteria can be helpful while others can be harmful to the body.
- **Immunosuppressant** - A medication that prevents or reduces the immune system's defensive actions that usually protect the body from invasion by foreign substances, such as bacteria and viruses; a type of medication often used by patients who have had organ transplants or certain diseases in which the immune system causes problems by attacking beneficial organs or tissues.
- **Infection** - Invasion of the body by a bacteria or virus.
- **Inflammation** - A localized response to injured tissue usually causing heat, pain, redness, and swelling.
- **Leukocyte** - A white blood cell which functions by fighting infections.

- **Pathogen** - A microorganism (bacteria or virus) that can cause a disease.
- **Virus** - A microorganism that invades body cells and replicates itself to eventually invade or spread to neighboring tissues.

Common Conditions and Diseases of the Lymphatic and Immune Systems

- **Acquired immunodeficiency syndrome (AIDS)** - A condition caused by infection by the human immunodeficiency virus (HIV). HIV infections progress into AIDS, which is characterized by severely compromised immunity. HIV is contagious and may be spread through body fluids such as blood and semen, often through unprotected sex or sharing IV needles.
- **Cellulitis** - Bacterial infection common on the legs usually caused by strep or staph infections.
- **Chickenpox** - A highly contagious acute viral disease characterized by fever and pustules on the skin.
- **Edema** - Also known as hypervolemia, in which an excessive amount of fluid accumulates in the body, often around the ankles. Ankle edema may be caused by heart failure.
- **Hepatitis A and E** - Inflammation of the liver caused by viruses usually acquired by consuming contaminated food or water.
- **Hepatitis B and C** - Inflammation of the liver caused by viruses usually acquired by unprotected sex, IV drug abuse or passed from the mother to child during pregnancy.
- **Human immunodeficiency virus (HIV)** - A pathogen that targets specific white blood cells (CD4 white blood cells) resulting in compromised immunity. Untreated HIV infections may lead to acquired immunodeficiency syndrome (AIDS).
- **Lymphoma** - Cancer in the lymph nodes which results in decreased immunity and increased susceptibility to infection.
- **Lupus-** An autoimmune disorder usually characterized by a decrease in blood cells, arthritis, and skin abnormalities especially on the face (butterfly rash).
- **Measles** - Highly contagious viral disease characterized by fever and small red spots with blue-white centers that appear on the skin and inside the mouth.
- **Mumps** - An acute viral disease characterized by swelling of the salivary glands.
- **Ringworm** - A type of fungal infection characterized by a raised red ring region on the skin.
- **Shingles** - A painful inflammation of nerve cells, usually on the trunk of the body, caused by the same virus that causes chicken pox, which may occur many years or decades after exposure to the virus.

The Digestive System

The alimentary canal, also called the gastrointestinal (GI) tract, is a long, muscular tube that twists and turns through the body digesting food and absorbing nutrients into the blood. The organs of the alimentary canal include the mouth, pharynx, esophagus, stomach, small intestine and large intestine. The large intestine leads to the anus, or opening at the end. Since the alimentary canal is open at both ends, technically, food material in the alimentary canal is considered outside of the body from the point of ingestion to defecation. The accessory digestive organs include the teeth, tongue, salivary glands, gallbladder, liver, and pancreas.

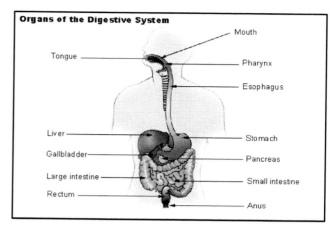

Food is ingested, and swallowed in the mouth. The pharynx, located in the throat, separates food from air and directs the food down the esophagus and into the stomach, located in the abdomen. The stomach is where most digestion takes place as food is churned and mixed with digestive enzymes from the liver, gallbladder, and pancreas that break it down and prepare it for absorption. Food then moves into the small intestine, located in the lower abdomen, which is the major site of absorption of vitamins, minerals, and water. Indigestible substances move into the large intestine, surrounding the small intestine in the lower abdomen, where they are dried, packed, and prepared for elimination. Peristalsis, contractions of the large intestine, ensures movement through the GI tract where the undigested material is expelled through the anus.

Common Terminology Associated with the Digestive System
- **Absorption** - Movement of a drug, nutrient, or water from the intestines into the circulatory system (or bloodstream).
- **ADME** – Acronym that describes how the drug moves into and out of the body. "A" stands for absorption, "D" stands for distribution, "M" stands for metabolism, and "E" stands for excretion.
- **Antiemetic** - A medication used for motion sickness that prevents or relieves nausea and vomiting.
- **Bile** - A fluid secreted by the liver that aids in the digestion of fats.
- **Colon** - The large intestine.
- **Colonoscopy** - Direct visual examination of the inner surface of the colon.
- **Digestion** - The breakdown and dissolving of food into smaller particles.
- **Distribution** – The process of carrying the drug through the body to its site of action.
- **Enter/o** - Intestine.
- **Excretion** – The process of expelling waste from the body by urination or defecation.

- **Gastr/o** - Stomach.
- **Hepat/o** - Liver.
- **Insulin** - Hormone secreted by the pancreas that aids in the digestion of sugar and maintenance of proper blood sugar level.
- **Laxative** - A medication used to stimulate elimination of waste products from the colon.
- **Metabolism** - A set of chemical reactions that occur within organisms in order to create energy and maintain tissues. Breaking down large molecules releases energy that is then used to build cells and proteins. Metabolism also breaks down chemicals or deactivates drugs. The liver is crucial for metabolism.
- **Or/o** - Mouth.
- **Peristalsis** - Contractions of the smooth muscle in the GI tract that propel or move food down the GI tract.
- **Sublingual** - Under the tongue.

Common Conditions and Diseases of the Digestive System
- **Cirrhosis** - A hardening of the liver caused by alcohol abuse and hepatitis.
- **Colon cancer** – Tumor growth in the colon. Patients should be screened for colon cancer by having a colonoscopy every 10 years starting at age 50 (earlier and more often if the patient has a higher risk.)
- **Constipation** - A condition in which the colon has difficulty eliminating waste products.
- **Diarrhea** - Abnormal frequency of loose or watery discharge from the colon that can result in dehydration
- **Diabetes** – A condition characterized by impaired metabolism and excessively high blood sugar, usually caused by insufficient production of insulin by the pancreas or abnormal resistance to insulin's effects. Diabetes may be seen in children (Type I) and obese adults (Type II). The symptoms of diabetes are excessive urination, thirst, and increased appetite. Acute reactions can result in altered consciousness or coma. Long-term complications can affect vision and blood circulation and can result in blindness, loss of circulation to the limbs and kidney failure.
- **Hepatitis** - Inflammation of the liver caused by viruses, bacterial infections, continuous exposure to alcohol or drugs, or an autoimmune disorders often resulting in compromised or decreased immunity.
- **Hyperglycemia** - An abnormally high concentration of sugar in the blood.
- **Hypoglycemia** - An abnormally low concentration of sugar in the blood.
- **Hyperlipidemia** – Excessive amount of fats in the blood; also known as high cholesterol, which can clog blood vessels, especially those of the heart.
- **Irritable Bowel Syndrome (IBS)** - A condition characterized by muscle spasms in the intestines and abdominal pain and may be accompanied by constipation or diarrhea.
- **Renal disease** – Disease pertaining to the kidneys, often seen in patients with diabetes or uncontrolled high blood pressure.
- **Ulcers** - Open sores or lesions in the GI tract, usually in the stomach or intestines, that result in pain, inflammation, and/or bleeding.

The Urinary System

The urinary system consists of the kidneys, urinary bladder, ureters and urethra. These organs function to eliminate waste products and conserve nutrients.

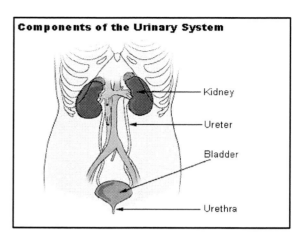

The kidneys are the major excretory organs in the body. They filter out toxins and metabolic waste from the blood and excrete them while returning essential substances back to the bloodstream. The kidneys contain millions of nephrons which produce about half a gallon of urine per day. Urine is transported from the kidneys to the urinary bladder in slender tubes called ureters. An empty, collapsed bladder is shaped like a pyramid. As the bladder fills with urine, the walls and surrounding muscles are stretched into the shape of a pear. This is the body's urine storage tank until release of urine is convenient. A moderately full bladder holds about one pint of urine. Urine is excreted from the body through the urethra. The length of the urethra is shorter in females than in males, which makes females more prone to urinary tract infections. In males, the urethra has a double function of carrying semen as well as urine out of the body.

Common Terminology Associated with the Urinary System
- **Ren/o, ren/i** - Kidney
- **Renal** - Pertaining to the kidney.
- **Uresis, -uresis** - Urination; excretion in urine.
- **Urinalysis** - The examination of the urine to determine the presence of certain substances, such as sugar levels, blood, etc.

Common Conditions and Diseases of the Urinary System
- **Benign Prostate Hyperplasia (BPH)** – Enlarged prostate gland, which can inhibit proper flow of urine.
- **Chronic renal failure** - A condition where the kidney is unable to clear or filter the blood properly.
- **Cystitis** - Inflammation of the urinary bladder caused by infection; resulting in the increased urge to urinate and burning sensation upon urinating.
- **Kidney stones** - Crystals that develop in the kidney, ureter, or urethra composed of calcium, uric acid, and other compounds causing difficulty urinating, blood in the urine and extreme pain.
- **Prostate cancer** – Tumor growth in the prostate gland usually characterized by difficulty urinating. Men should begin screening every year at age 50 (unless at high risk.)

- **Urethritis** - Inflammation of the urethra which causes a burning sensation during urination.
- **Urinary tract infection (UTI)** - Infection of any part of the urinary tract, usually the urethra and urinary bladder; caused by bacteria.

The Nervous System

The nervous system regulates and coordinates the various systems of the body and helps the body to adjust to changes in the environment. The nervous system can be divided into two parts: the central nervous system (CNS) and the peripheral nervous system (PNS). The CNS consists of the brain and spinal cord where information is gathered and interpreted, and where voluntary muscle movements and other body functions are initiated. The PNS lies outside of the CNS and links the rest of the body to the central nervous system through a network of nerves that carry impulses to and from the brain and spinal cord. Sensory nerve fibers transmit impulses to the CNS from the skin, skeletal muscles and organs. Motor nerve fibers convey impulses from the CNS to the rest of the body. The PNS is further divided into two groups: (1) the somatic nervous system, commonly called the voluntary nervous system, which controls conscious muscle movement and (2) the autonomic nervous system (ANS) which directs involuntary activities such as the beating of our hearts and digestion.

Common Terminology Associated with the Nervous System
- **Anesthetic** - A medication which decreases the body's sensitivity to pain or touch.
- **Anticonvulsant** - A medication designed to prevent seizures or convulsions.
- **Antidepressant** - A medication designed to prevent or relieve depression.
- **Antipsychotic** - A medication used to treat severe psychiatric disorders.
- **Barbiturate** - A medication class which depresses the CNS, resulting in calmness or sleep.
- **Cephal/o** - Head.
- **Cerebrospinal fluid (CSF)** - A clear, watery fluid produced by the brain that helps cushion the brain and the spinal cord from injury.
- **Electroencephalography (EEG)** - The process of making graphs of the electrical activity of the brain.
- **Encephal/o** - Brain.
- **Neuropathy** - Any disease of the nervous system.
- **Nerv/o, Nerv/i, Neur/o, Neur/i** - Nerve.
- **Nerve** - Composed of neurons that connect the brain or spinal cord to other parts of the body.
- **Neuron** - A specialized impulse-conducting cell that is the functional unit of the nervous system which forms nerves.
- **Sedative** - A medication which depresses the CNS resulting in calmness or sleep.
- **Stimulus** - Anything that excites or activates a nerve.

Common Conditions and Diseases of the Nervous System

- **Alzheimer's disease** - A group of disorders associated with brain degeneration leading to progressive memory loss and personality changes.
- **Attention deficit hyperactive disorder (ADHD)** - A behavior disorder usually in young children characterized by inattentiveness, hyperactivity, and impulsiveness.
- **Bipolar disorder** - A condition characterized by irregular, alternating periods of mania and depression.
- **Coma** - A prolonged state of unconsciousness with no response to stimuli.
- **Dementia** - Slow, progressive deterioration of brain affecting everyday activities such as memory, thinking, alertness, and reasoning.
- **Depression** – A mood disorder characterized by a lack of cheerfulness, dejection, loss of hope and lack of interest in daily activities.
- **Insomnia** - A condition characterized by the inability to sleep; usually caused by depression, pain, or excessive caffeine intake.
- **Mania** - A mental state characterized by excessive excitement and feelings of grandeur.
- **Meningitis** - Inflammation of the membranes covering the central nervous system (i.e., brain and spinal cord) characterized by neck stiffness, headache, altered mental status, and fever usually caused by bacteria.
- **Multiple sclerosis (MS)** - Chronic, progressive degeneration of the central nervous system that can result in decreased stimulation, paralysis, shakiness, and speech abnormalities.
- **Narcolepsy** - Syndrome characterized by uncontrolled drowsiness and sleepiness.
- **Obsessive-compulsive disorder (OCD)** - A condition characterized by persistent ideas, thoughts, or images causing anxiety and distress along with corresponding behaviors designed to reduce anxiety or stress, such as repeated hand-washing.
- **Parkinson's disease** - A progressive, degenerative central nervous system disorder characterized by constant muscle spasms and shakiness.
- **Posttraumatic stress disorder (PTSD)** - A condition characterized by anxiety, depression, difficulty concentrating, restlessness, and sleep disorders caused by a previous traumatic event such as experiencing or witnessing violence.
- **Schizophrenia** - A psychotic disorder characterized by separation from reality usually accompanied by abnormal behavior, illogical thinking, and hallucinations.
- **Stroke** - Damage to the brain caused by either a blockage of blood supply to the brain or a hemorrhage in the brain; also known as a cerebrovascular accident (CVA).

The Integumentary (Skin) System

The skin, sweat and oil glands, hair, and nails make up the integumentary system. The primary function of the integumentary system is to protect the internal organs and tissues from pathogens and the environment but it also serves to regulate body temperature, perceive stimuli and serve as a blood reserve. The skin is the covering of the body and its first-line barrier against bacteria and viruses as well as to decrease the loss of water. The skin consists of two distinct layers: the epidermis and the dermis. The epidermis is the upper surface where tightly connected, protein-filled cells are produced giving the skin its continuity and suppleness. It is thicker in "contact" areas (the palms of the hands, fingertips, and soles of the feet) and thinner over the rest of the body. As these cells die, they are sloughed off by the millions each day and replaced. The skin may also contain a pigment, known as melanin, for protection from the sun's ultraviolet (UV) rays. Specialized cells from the immune system are also present in the epidermis to help thwart viral and bacterial invasions. Below the epidermis is another elastic, fibrous tissue called the dermis. The dermis houses sensory receptors, blood vessels, oil and sweat glands, and hair follicles. The strong and flexible fibers of the dermis provide durability and resilience.

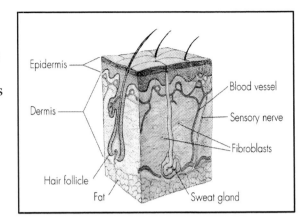

Sweat glands continually secrete an unnoticeable amount of sweat when the environmental temperature is mild and the body is resting. When the internal or external temperature rises, blood vessels in the dermis dilate and sweat glands are stimulated to increase the output of sweat, which cools the body when it evaporates. If the air outside is cold, the blood vessels constrict, warm blood bypasses the skin, and internal heat is conserved. Hair on our heads helps protect us from heat loss, head trauma and sunlight. Eyelashes protect our eyes from the sun and nose hair filters incoming air. Body hair is designed to sense insects on the skin before they can sting or bite!

Common Terminology Associated with the Integumentary System

- **Derm/a, Derm/o, Dermat/o, -derma** - Skin
- **Diaphoresis** - Excessive sweating
- **Perspiration** - Sweating
- **Subcutaneous** - The layer below the cutaneous (dermal) skin layer and a common location for injections
- **Topical** - A medication (usually a cream or ointment) applied to a localized area on a body surface
- **Transdermal** - A medication applied to the skin such as a nitroglycerin or nicotine patch

Common Conditions and Diseases of the Integumentary System

- **Burn** - Tissue damage resulting from excessive exposure of the skin to heat, chemicals or radiation. Burns can be classified according to the extent of tissue damage:
  - 1st degree - A superficial burn limited to the outer layer of the epidermis. Lighter-skinned individuals will show redness as with a sunburn.
  - 2nd degree - A burn that penetrates the epidermis and into the dermis but not so severely that it inhibits regeneration of the epidermis. Second-degree burns are characterized by blisters.
  - 3rd degree - A burn in which all of the epidermis and dermis are destroyed.
- **Contusion** - An injury in which tissues or blood vessels or damaged but does not break the skin; a bruise.
- **Contact dermatitis** - Inflammation of the skin characterized by redness and itching caused by contact with an irritant or allergen.
- **Eczema (atopic dermatitis)** - An acute or chronic skin inflammation characterized by redness, inflammation, scales, scabs, and itching.
- **Gangrene** - Tissue death followed by bacterial infection resulting in foul-smelling decayed sores.
- **Hives** - A condition in which the skin reacts to allergens or stress by developing round elevations with red edges and pale centers.
- **Impetigo** - A contagious bacterial infection that is common in children that results in red lesions, usually around the face and hands
- **Laceration** - A cut or tear in the skin.
- **Melanoma** - A form or skin cancer that may result from excessive exposure to the sun.
- **Pruritis** - Itching.
- **Psoriasis** - Metabolic skin disorder where the skin has red raised rashes with white to silver scales caused by accelerated growth of skin cells.
- **Septic shock** – Severe complication of an infection resulting in organ dysfunction and abnormally low blood pressure; often resulting in severe shock or sudden death.
- **Tinea pedis (athlete's foot)** - Highly contagious fungal infection on feet and between toes characterized by dry and crusty areas of skin.
- **Wart** – An elevated growth on the skin caused by a virus.

The Endocrine System

The endocrine system is a group of glands and organs that release hormones to control various bodily functions such as cellular metabolism, reproduction, growth and development, and electrolyte balance. A hormone is a chemical messenger released into the blood stream that regulates the functions of other cells. The major endocrine glands of the body consist of the pineal, pituitary, thyroid, parathyroid, thymus, and adrenal glands. Endocrine organs include the pancreas and the gonads (testes, in males and ovaries, in females).

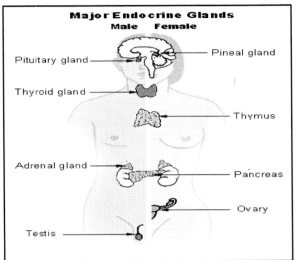

The pineal gland, located in the brain, secretes melatonin, which increases in the blood at night and makes us drowsy and falls during daylight hours.

The pituitary gland is also located in the brain and secretes a number of hormones which regulate various body functions including growth, reproduction and some metabolic functions.

The butterfly-shaped thyroid gland is located in the neck and releases thyroid hormone, which is the body's major metabolic hormone. Thyroid hormone regulates body temperature, appetite, weight, and blood pressure.

The four parathyroid glands are located on the thyroid gland and secrete parathyroid hormone, regulating calcium balance in the blood.

The thymus, located in the chest, promotes the maturity of lymphocytes, thus playing and important role in immune system function.

The pancreas, located in the abdomen, releases glucagon and insulin to raise and lower blood sugar, respectively.

The adrenal glands are located on top of the kidneys. They secrete aldosterone, cortisol (hydrocortisone), testosterone, epinephrine and norepinephrine. Aldosterone regulates sodium and water levels; cortisol helps the body resist stressors; testosterone contributes to the onset of puberty and the development of pubic hair; and epinephrine and norepinephrine promote the "fight or flight" effects in response to emergency situations.

The male and female gonads produce sex hormones. Female ovaries produce estrogen and progesterone promoting breast development, egg production and the menstrual cycle. Male testes produce testosterone promoting sperm production and libido.

215

Common Terminology Associated with the Endocrine System

- **Hydrocortisone -** A synthetic hormone used to relieve or reduce inflammation, pain, and organ rejection.
- **Steroid -** A term describing certain sex hormones and hormones produced by the adrenal glands. Steroids can be natural or synthetic and are used to treat a wide variety of conditions.

Common Conditions and Diseases of the Endocrine System

- **Goiter -** The abnormal development of the thyroid gland resulting in an enlargement in the frontal part of the neck.
- **Hyperglycemia -** A condition characterized by abnormally high levels of sugar in the blood, as in diabetes. Hyperglycemia can increase susceptibility to infections and result in diabetic coma.
- **Hypoglycemia -** A condition characterized by abnormally low levels of sugar in the blood resulting in weakness, fatigue and irritability and possibly hypoglycemic coma.
- **Hyperparathyroidism -** A condition characterized by abnormally high levels of parathyroid hormone in the body resulting in weak bones.
- **Hypoparathyroidism -** A condition characterized by abnormally low levels of parathyroid hormone in the body resulting in cramps.
- **Hyperthyroidism -** A condition characterized by excessive thyroid hormone levels in the body resulting in increased sweating, nervousness, and weight loss.
- **Hypothyroidism -** A condition characterized by deficient amounts of thyroid hormone levels resulting in fatigue, depression, and weight gain.

The Reproductive System

The reproductive system is the only system that is not required for the survival of an individual. However, the reproductive system is necessary for the survival of a species. The primary organs of the reproductive system are called gonads. The gonads produce gametes, or sex cells. The male gonads are called testes and the female gonads are called ovaries. The male gametes are called sperm and the female gametes are called eggs or ova.

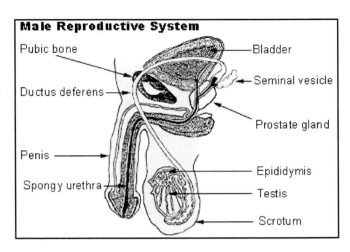

Reproduction can occur when sperm fertilizes an ovum as it passes through the fallopian tubes. After fertilization, the ovum (now called a zygote) is transported to the uterus. Once the zygote implants into the uterus it is referred to as an embryo. Between the ninth week of pregnancy until the time of birth, the developing embryo is referred to as a fetus.

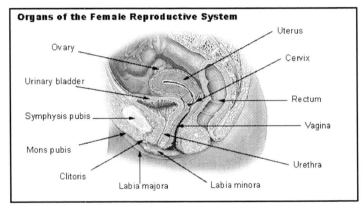

Common Terminology Associated with the Reproductive System

- **Amenorhea** – The absence of a menstrual period in women between puberty and menopause.
- **Cesarean delivery (C-section)** – Delivery of a baby by making an incision in the pregnant mother's abdominal and uterine wall.
- **Fallopian tubes** – Tubes in females where fertilization of the egg occurs.
- **Gynec** - female
- **Gynecologist** – A specialist in diagnosing and treating disorders of the female reproductive system.
- **Menopause** – The stopping of menstruation.
- **Menstruation** – The normal periodic (usually monthly) shedding of bloody fluid and discharge from the non-pregnant uterus, also know as menses.
- **Oral contraceptive** – Tablets taken by mouth which prevent pregnancy; also known as birth control pills.
- **Ova** – The female gametes; also known as egg cells.
- **Ovary** – Female reproductive organ that produces eggs and secretes estrogen and progesterone.
- **Ovulation** – The release of an egg every month by the ovary.

- **Penis** – Male sex organ that delivers sperm into female vagina.
- **Placenta** – An organ that develops between a mother and fetus during pregnancy where nutrients and waste are exchanged.
- **Prostate** – Gland found in males that secretes lubricant during ejaculation.
- **Testicle** – Male reproductive gland that produces sperm and testosterone.
- **Urethra** – A tube found in males that passes through the penis that functions in urination and reproduction.
- **Uterus** – An organ in females that protects and supports the developing fetus.
- **Vagina** – Female muscular tube that accepts the male penis; also known as the birth canal.

Common Conditions and Diseases of the Reproductive System

- **Acquired immunodeficiency syndrome (AIDS)** - A condition caused by HIV which describes the later stages of infection characterized by severely compromised immunity. HIV can be transmitted sexually.
- **Breast cancer** – Tumor growth in breast tissue, usually in females. Women should be screened for breast cancer by having a monthly breast self exam starting at age 20, a clinical breast exam every 3 years between the ages of 20 and 30 and every year beginning at age 40, and a mammogram every year starting at age 40 (more often for patients who are at high risk).
- **Chlamydia** – A highly contagious sexually transmitted infection caused by a bacteria and resulting in damage to reproductive organs if not treated early.
- **Erectile Dysfunction (ED)** – The inability of a male to obtain or maintain an erection; also known as impotence.
- **Genital Herpes** – A sexually transmitted disease caused by a virus; characterized by painful blisters on genitals. Genital herpes cannot be cured but symptoms may be treated.
- **Gonorrhea** – A sexually transmitted disease caused by a bacterium; characterized by a burning or painful sensation while urinating, vaginal or penile discharge, and sore throat.
- **Human immunodeficiency virus (HIV)** - A sexually transmitted disease that targets specific white blood cells (CD4 white blood cells) resulting in compromised immunity.
- **Sexual Transmitted Infection (STI)** – Infections transmitted by sexual contact. Also called STD, or, sexually transmitted disease.
- **Syphilis** – An STI caused by a bacterium characterized by painless sores, swollen lymph nodes, fever, fatigue, and loss of appetite.
- **Trichomoniasis** – An STI caused by a protozoan characterized by pain during sexual intercourse, vaginal or penile discharge, and itching.

SELF-ASSESSMENT QUESTIONS CHAPTER XII

1. Which of the following best describes the function of the cardiovascular system?
   a. Transports oxygen and nutrients to the organs and tissues of the body.
   b. Protects the body from bacterial and viral infection, allergic reactions, and tumors.
   c. Brings oxygen into the body while releasing carbon dioxide from the body.
   d. Senses, interprets, and responds to stimuli in order to maintain normal function or homeostasis.

2. Which of the following is another name for a cerebrovascular accident?
   a. Stroke
   b. Heart attack
   c. Asthma attack
   d. Acid reflux

3. The ingestion, absorption, and excretion of foods and nutrients is best characterized by which of the following systems?
   a. Digestive system.
   b. Nervous system.
   c. Integumentary system
   d. Endocrine system

4. Which of the following conditions is best characterized by the inability to sleep usually caused by depression, pain, or excessive caffeine intake?
   a. Narcolepsy
   b. Insomnia
   c. Dementia
   d. Amnesia

5. Which of the following best describes the function of a leukocyte?
   a. Blood vessel that carries deoxygenated blood towards the heart.
   b. Blood vessel that carries oxygenated blood away from the heart.
   c. One of numerous sites throughout the body where oxygen is exchanged from the red blood cells to the body organs and tissues.
   d. Blood cell, which functions by fighting infections.

Answers:
1) a
2) a
3) a
4) b
5) d

PHARMACY TECHNICIAN COMPETENCY ASSESSMENT

CHAPTER XII

Description of Ability or Skill	Initials		Training Completed	
	Tech	R.Ph.	Date	Remarks
The technician trainee can properly identify basic anatomical structures.				
The technician trainee properly uses basic medical terminology.				
The technician trainee can define common medical conditions.				

Photo sources:
- digestive, respiratory, urinary, endocrine systems
  http://training.seer.cancer.gov/module_anatomy/unit1_1_body_structure.html
  date accessed: March 1, 2007
- immune system
  http://www.niaid.nih.gov/final/immun/immun.htm
  date accessed: March 1, 2007
- skin
  http://publications.nigms.nih.gov/factsheets/artificialskin.html
  date accessed: March 1, 2007

Chapter XIII
Over-the-Counter (OTC) Medications
By: Brandon M. Williams

EDUCATIONAL OBJECTIVES
After studying the material in this chapter, the technician trainee should be able to: • List the major OTC categories and subcategories. • Identify the condition that a given OTC product is designed to treat. • Identify the generic and brand-names of commonly used OTC medications. • Identify the functions that pharmacy technicians may and may not perform with regard to OTC medications. • Identify medications that should be avoided by patients with certain conditions such as high blood pressure and diabetes. • Recognize which OTC products require a patient to sign a Schedule V sales log • Identify the major functions of various vitamins and minerals. • Be able to find information regarding herbal medications

As a pharmacy technician, your duties may not be limited to the prescription counter. Often, patients will ask you to help them find over-the-counter (OTC) medications outside the pharmacy department. The retail space surrounding your pharmacy department contains many health and beauty care products. Health aids include such products as vitamins, pain relievers, and antacids. Beauty aids include products such as shampoos, conditioners, skin creams, and after-shave lotions.

Medications are granted over-the-counter status only when the Food and Drug Administration is satisfied that they can be used safely without the supervision of a prescriber. All information for safe and effective use must be printed on the package and items that could be harmful to children must be packaged in child-resistant containers.

Your pharmacy may stock many different types of OTC medications. Once you understand how these products have been organized, you should not have trouble locating specific products. Each store has several OTC categories, such as cough and cold products, analgesics, antacids, laxatives, etc. Each category may have several subcategories. For example, the cough and cold products category includes: cough syrups, allergy products, asthma remedies, etc. Each subcategory is composed of a group of better-selling brands. Within the brands are the better-selling package sizes and dosage forms. In many cases, generic and "private label" versions (i.e., generic equivalents bearing your pharmacy's name on the package) of these medications may be displayed next to the brand name.

OUTLINE OF OTC CATEGORIES AND SUBCATEGORIES

Many pharmacy departments have signs posted in the aisles to help patients find specific product categories. However, people often times do not know the category to which a particular product belongs, so they are likely to ask you. Thus, you should know where various OTC products are located in the pharmacy. Hunting for a product increases patient frustration, so when patients ask you where to find an item, do not merely point to an area and say, "It's over there in Aisle 3." Delivering good patient service means you give clear directions or escort patients to the shelf and show them the product.

> **Note:** Always be helpful, but provide information that is within your limits. Any questions about ingredients, medication interactions, or side effects must be referred to a pharmacist. You may relay a pharmacist's answers but **you should not answer the questions yourself nor should you recommend a specific product.**

OTC products can be used to treat a wide variety of self-limiting conditions and minor symptoms such as fever, cough, sneezing, stuffy nose, allergies, headaches, cold sores, motion sickness, etc. Products approved by the FDA for sale over the counter must have labels and directions that are clear enough for patients to understand the products' indications, dosages, and potential problems. OTC products can pose problems for patients who may unwittingly take medication that duplicates or interacts with other medications that they are taking or is contraindicated for them. While pharmacy technicians cannot recommend these products, they can encourage patients to ask the pharmacist for advice or remind patients to carefully read the package labeling. A table outlining the names and uses of common over-the-counter medications is included at the end of this chapter.

Following is a description of some of the most common categories of over-the-counter products.

Analgesics (pain relievers)

- **Internal analgesics** are taken orally to relieve pain such as headache, toothache, menstrual cramps and joint aches. Some analgesics, like aspirin and ibuprofen, also reduce fever and inflammation. Aspirin, acetaminophen (Tylenol®) and non-steroidal anti-inflammatory drugs (NSAIDs) are commonly used. Ibuprofen is an example of an NSAID. Generally, aspirin should be avoided children. Because of their effects on blood platelets, aspirin and NSAIDs should be avoided if the patient shows symptoms and signs of bleeding. Acetaminophen use should be monitored very closely to limit dosage below 4g (4,000mg) per day as overdose can result in irreversible liver damage or even death. However, acetaminophen may be an appropriate analgesic choice for patients who have gastric ulcers or high blood pressure. Due to the risk of Reye's syndrome, aspirin should NOT be given in children less than 14 years old with fever or cold. Instead, acetaminophen should be given to children less than 14 years old.
- **External analgesics** are applied topically to relieve the ache of minor sprains, strains, muscle aches, joint pain, and the pain and itching of hemorrhoids. Several medications used to treat muscle aches and pain include methyl salicylate (Icy Hot® or Thera-gesic®), trolamine salicylate (Aspercream®), and capsaicin (Zostrix®). Pramoxine (Preparation-H®) is an example of a product used to relieve pain and itching from hemorrhoids.

Antacids/Laxatives

- **Antacids** reduce stomach acid and can be used to treat the symptoms of gastroesophogeal reflux disease (GERD), or heartburn, and give temporary relief from ulcers. Calcium carbonate (TUMS®), magnesium hydroxide (Mylanta®), and sodium bicarbonate (Alka-seltzer®) are generally used first for heartburn. If heartburn is not relieved, ranitidine (Zantac®) or famotidine (Pepcid AC®) may be used. For severe heartburn or GERD, omeprazole (Prilosec OTC®) or higher doses of ranitidine (Zantac®) or famotidine (Pepcid AC®) may be used. Also note that there are prescription-only strengths of many of these medications.
- **Anti-flatulents** reduce discomfort of gas in stomach or intestines. Alpha-galactosidase (Beano®) is often used with meals that often trigger gas production. Beano® does not eliminate gas production already present but instead aids digestion by reducing or preventing future gas production. Simethicone (Gas-X®) is used to eliminate gas already present as well as reduce future gas production.
- **Laxatives** relieve constipation, correct incomplete or irregular bowel movements, or evacuate the bowel before rectal exams. Common laxatives include Metamucil®, Citrucel®, and Dulcolax®. There are also laxatives that are dispensed only by prescription.
- **Anti-diarrheals** reduce or stop diarrhea. Loperamide (Imodium®), and bismuth subsalicylate (Pepto-Bismol®) are often used. If a patient has diarrhea with flatulence, Imodium AD® may be used because Imodium AD® also contains simethicone. Due to the

risk of Reye's syndrome, Pepto-bismol® or Kaopectate® should NOT be given in children less than 14 years old with fever or cold. Instead, loperamide (Imodium®) may be given to children less than 14 years old if taken according to package directions.

Cough & Cold

- **Cough syrups** soothe the throat, suppress coughs or act as an expectorant to loosen phlegm in the respiratory tract. For productive cough (cough with mucus), an expectorant such as guaifenesin (Robitussin®) may be used. For a non-productive, dry hacking cough, dextromethorphan (Delsym®) may be used. Patients with diabetes should avoid syrups with a high sugar content and instead use sugar-free syrups or sugar-free cough drops for sore throat and cough. Robitussin AC® and a few other antitussive products contain codeine and are Schedule V Controlled Substances, which are available without a prescription in most states. Consequently, they are stored behind the counter.

- **Cold tablets, capsules, and liquids** are usually a combination of two or more active ingredients used to dry a runny nose or reduce nasal congestion; they may also contain pain relievers to reduce aches and fever. Many cold medication combos include an analgesic such as acetaminophen, an antihistamine such as diphenhydramine, a nasal decongestant such as phenyephrine, and a cough suppressant such as dextromethorphan. Products containing nasal decogestants such as pseudoepherdrine or phenylephrine should be avoided in patients with high blood pressure. Products containing antihistamines such as Benadryl® may cause drowsiness and should be avoided in patients who plan to drive or operate machinery.

- **Allergy products** reduce the itching, runny nose, swelling, and inflammation of minor allergic reactions. Diphenhydramine (Benadryl®), certirizine (Zyrtec®), and loratadine (Claritin®) are often used for allergies. Certirizine and loratadine are less sedating than diphenhydramine. Loratadine is used to treat runny noses due allergies whereas diphenhydramine can be used for a runny nose related to allergies as well as colds. However, diphenhydramine is highly sedating and should not be used when driving or operating machinery.

- **Nasal sprays, drops, and inhalers** reduce nasal congestion by reducing swelling of nasal tissues. Levmetamfetamine (Vicks Vapor Rub®) inhaler and oxymetazoline (Afrin®) nasal spray are common topical nasal degongestants used. Nasal decongestants such as oxymetazoline (Afrin®) or phenylephrine (Neo-Synephrine®) should be used for no more than three days. If used longer, symptoms may come back worse than before because of an effect known as rebound congestion.

- **Throat lozenges, sprays, and cough drops** relieve sore throat and minor coughs. Cepacol® lozenges and Halls® cough drops are examples of products that are used for sore throat.

- **Lip preparations** may treat cold sores and soothe chapped lips. Docosanol (Abreva®) is used for cold sores.

Eye/Ear

- **General eye care** products may relieve stinging, itching, dryness, or redness. A variety of products are available for eye irritation. Clear Eyes® and Visine® are commonly used eye drops. Several eye drop products contain a topical decongestant and an antihistamine. Decongestants should be used for no more than three days. A relatively new OTC product, ketotifen (Alaway® or Zaditor®), is an eye drop that contains an antihistamine without a decongestant. Ketotifen may be used to relieve itching of the eye due to allergies. Ketotifen may also be used longer than three days if approved by a physician.
- **Contact lens care** products include lens cleansers, disinfectants, rinses, and storage containers.
- **Ear-drying agents** remove water in the outer ear canal to prevent a painful condition known as "swimmer's ear." These products usually contain isopropyl alcohol (isopropanol). Examples are Auro-Dri®, SwimEar® and StarOtic®.
- **Softening agents** soften ear wax, which may then be flushed out of the ear. Carbamide peroxide (Debrox® or Murine®) are examples of ear wax removal products. Patients should avoid using Q-tips®, which may push ear wax deeper into the ear and worsen hearing.

First Aid

- **Antiseptics** kill germs and keep wounds from getting infected. Isopropyl alcohol is a commonly used antiseptic used in minor cuts and scrapes.
- **Antibiotic creams and ointments.** Neosporin® and Polysporin® are topical antibiotics that are used to to prevent infections from developing in minor cuts and scrapes. Neosporin® contains neomycin, to which some patients may be allergic. If a patient is allergic to neomycin, Polysporin® may be used instead.
- **Anesthetic creams and ointments** treat irritating and itchy rashes, insect bites, stings, and sunburn. Itch-X® is an anesthetic that contains pramoxine and benzyl alcohol and is commonly used to prevent itching from insect bites or stings. Benzocaine (Lanacane®) and lidocaine (Bactine®) may also be used for insect bites and stings.
- **Pediculocides** are used to kill lice. The most common product is lindane shampoo, which is sold as Kwell® Shampoo and Scabene® Shampoo. These products kill lice and their eggs but do not prevent infestations. The product is poisonous and must only be used topically. As with all OTC products, it is important to follow the directions carefully.
- **Antifungals** include creams, ointments, powders and sprays that treat fungal infections such as ringworm, jock itch, and athlete's foot. Clotrimazole (Lotrimin®), miconazole (Micatin®), terbinafine (Lamisil®), and butenafine (Lotrimin Ultra®) are commonly used for fungal infections.
- **Sunburn and burn products** usually contain a topical anesthetic such as lidocaine (Solarcaine®) that are used to relieve pain and itching. These products are supplied as sprays, gels, or creams.

- **Dry skin products** are usually supplied as creams or lotions. Examples are Lubriderm®, Eucerin®, and Vaseline Intensive Care Lotion®. Lotions contain various ingredients such as petrolatum, mineral oil, glycerin, propylene glycol, lecithin, and dimethicone, which moisturize the skin. Urea and lactic acid may also be added to improve penetration into the skin.
- **Poison ivy, oak, or sumac** products are topical anesthetics designed to relieve itching. Calamine lotion is an old remedy used for poison ivy, oak, or sumac that tends to dry out and flake off the skin a short time after application. There are numerous other remedies, such as pramoxine (Itch-X®), that are commonly used to relieve itching caused by poison ivy, oak, or sumac. Calamine lotion may also be used for poison ivy, oak, or sumac.

Foot Care

- **Antifungals** for the treatment of athlete's foot are often stocked in the foot-care section as well as the first-aid section. (See the previous discussion of antifungals.) These products are often supplied as sprays, creams or powders. Powders have the advantage of helping to keep feet dry, which can help prevent athlete's foot but they do not stay in contact with the skin as long as creams.
- **Foot discomfort aids** may be used to treat corns, calluses, bunions, ingrown toenails, and warts. Some of these products involve medications, such as salicylic acid (CompoundW®), which is commonly used to treat warts located on the hands and feet. However, these products should not be used for genital warts. There are also OTC wart removers which freeze off warts but these are more expensive. Other non-drug products include pads, cushions and arch supports. The latter are commonly used to relieve heel pain (plantar fasciitis).

Home Health Care

- **Convalescent aids** include canes, crutches, bed pans, cervical collars, etc.
- **Durable medical equipment** include "durable," long-lasting patient aids, such as wheel-chairs, crutches, canes, walkers, and hospital beds. It is important that patients adjust crutches and walkers to the proper height.
- **Other home health care products** include ostomy supplies, wound management supplies, incontinence aids, vaporizers, etc.

Motion Sickness

- **Motion sickness remedies** relieve nausea and vomiting due to motion sickness. Meclizine (Dramamine Less Drowsy®), dimenhydinate (Dramamine®), and diphenhydramine (Benadryl®) are common examples. Products other than meclizine tend to cause drowsiness and should be avoided by patients who intend to drive or operating machinery.

Self-Testing

- **Blood-glucose meters** measure the concentration of sugar in the blood. People with diabetes measure their blood-sugar levels by drawing a drop of blood from their finger with a device called a "lancet". The blood is placed on a test strip or on a drum in which the blood-sugar level is then read by the meter.
- **Blood pressure monitors** may be manual or automatic and arm or wrist blood pressure devices. Many community pharmacies also have automatic arm blood pressure devices that patient can use at the pharmacy. To get an accurate reading, the patient should sit still for a minute or two before taking a reading.
- **Monitoring accessories** include alcohol, cotton balls, alcohol wipes, and test strips.
- **Syringes** are used for insulin and other injections and may be stored behind the pharmacy department counter. Syringes come in many sizes with some being made only for insulin administration. Some states require that records be kept of those people who purchase needles and/or syringes.
- **Home test kits** measure the concentration of sugar in the blood or in the urine, blood cholesterol levels, ovulation and pregnancy, etc. Patients should follow the directions carefully and report their results to their physician.

Sleep Aids

- **Sleep aids** cause drowsiness, allowing patients to fall asleep more easily. Some of these products, such as Benadryl® (diphenhydramine), are actually antihistamines, which are used for treatment of allergies. Since a common side effect of these products is drowsiness, patients can also take them as a sleep aids. Obviously, patients should not use these medications before driving or operating machinery. They should also be cautious about consuming alcohol with these products as the combination of alcohol and antihistamines can increase the sedative effect.

Supplements

- **Vitamins** are essential substances needed to perform everyday functions. Although appropriate levels of vitamins can be achieved through a normal diet, there are cases in which patients may have vitamin deficiencies that can be treated with a vitamin supplement. Contrary to popular belief, vitamins do not necessarily give individual more energy or stamina. Vitamins are classified into two main categories: fat-soluble and water-soluble. Fat-soluble vitamins are deposited in fat cells and can be toxic in high doses. Water-soluble vitamins, on the other hand, are used by the body as needed and any excess supply is excreted through the urine. A table at the end of this chapter outlines some of the uses for various vitamins.
- **Dietary minerals** are chemical elements other than the four elements carbon, hydrogen, oxygen and nitrogen that are present in organic compounds and are essential for maintaining biological functions and normal metabolism. The most well-known minerals are calcium and iron. Although appropriate intake of minerals is necessary for optimum health, this level is usually achieved with a healthy diet. A table at the end of this chapter outlines some of the uses of some of the more common dietary minerals.

- **Herbal remedies** are traditional or folk medicines based on the use of plants and plant extracts. Herbal medicines may also include certain natural fungi, bee products, animal parts, shells and minerals. Hundreds of herbal remedies are advertised for treatment of a wide variety of symptoms including chondroitin sulfate, echinacea, ephedra, garlic, ginkgo biloba, ginseng, glucosamine, kava, melatonin, black cohosh, saw palmetto and St. John's wort. Some individuals may see herbal remedies as preferable alternatives to industrially produced chemical medications. The FDA, however, does not regulate herbal products because they are considered "nutritional supplements" rather than drugs. It is very important to understand that herbal remedies are not always proven to be effective and can interact with other medications.

Vitamins

Fat-soluble vitamins		
Vitamin	**Scientific Name**	**Functions**
Vitamin A	Retinol (beta-carotene)	Essential in bone and tooth development.
Vitamin D	Ergocalciferol	Increases calcium absorption.
Vitamin E	Alpha-tocopherol	Used as an antioxidant. (Antioxidants protect the body from substances that can damage the cells.)
Vitamin K[*]	Phytonadione	Helps in proper clotting of the blood.

Water-soluble vitamins		
Vitamin	**Scientific Name**	**Functions**
Vitamin B1	Thiamine	Supports proper function of nervous system.
Vitamin B2	Riboflavin	Promotes good vision and healthy skin.
Vitamin B3	Niacin	Helps digestion, promotes healthy skin and nerves and improves cholesterol levels.
Vitamin B5	Pantothenic Acid	Promotes formation of hormones.
Vitamin B6	Pyridoxine	Assists protein metabolism and red blood cell formation
Vitamin B7	Biotin	Aids fat synthesis.
Vitamin B9[**]	Folic Acid	Prevents brain and spinal birth defects.
Vitamin B12[***]	Cyanocobalamin	Maintains nervous system.
Vitamin C	Ascorbic Acid	Aids in wound healing. bone and tooth formation, and is vital for the function of the immune system.

[*]   Vitamin K is sometimes available OTC in small doses in combination with other vitamins; Vitamin K is available by itself only by prescription.
[**]   Folic acid (B9) is available OTC in doses of 800 mcg or less; higher doses require a prescription.
[***] Vitamin B12 is available OTC in a solid dosage form; the injectable form requires a prescription.

Dietary Minerals

Mineral	Functions
Calcium	Proper function of muscle, heart, digestive system, bones, blood cells
Fluorine	Formation of tooth enamel
Iodine	Proper function of the thyroid gland
Iron	Transport of oxygen by hemoglobin in red blood cells
Potassium	Proper function of Bones, muscles, metabolism and maintaining proper sodium levels
Sodium	Metabolism and maintaining proper potassium levels
Zinc	Proper function of certain enzymes

Herbal Products

Herbal products are available over-the-counter, and are not regulated be the FDA. Therefore, a product's active ingredient(s) may not be authentic or proven to work. An excellent reference for herbal medications is the *Natural Medicines Comprehensive Database* online (http://www.naturaldatabase.com). Ask the pharmacist if the pharmacy has a subscription to this online database. Listed below are some common herbal products.

Herbal Product	Condition Prevented / Treated	Effectiveness
Aloe vera	Wounds, burns	Unknown
Black Cohosh	Menopausal symptoms	Possibly
Caffeine	Headache, mental alertness	Headache (effective), mental alertness (possibly)
Chondroitin	Osteoarthritis, eye surgery	Eye surgery (likely), osetoarthritis (possibly)
Coenzyme Q10	Heart failure, blood pressure, heart attack	Possibly
Cranberry	Urinary tract infection	Possibly
Dong Quai	Premature ejaculation	Possibly
Echinacea	Common cold	Possibly
Evening Primrose Oil	Myalgia, osteoporosis	Possibly
Feverfew	Migraine headache	Possibly
Fish oil	High trigycerides	Effective
Ginko	Dementia, intermittent claudication	Possibly
Ginseng	Cognitive function	Possibly
Glucosamine sulfate	Osteoarthritis	Likely
Hoodia	Weight loss	Unknown
Kava kava	Anxiety	Possibly
Psyllium	Constipation	Effective
Red yeast rice	High cholesterol	Likely
SAMe	Osteoarthritis, depression	Likely
Saw Palmetto	Benign prostate hyperplasia (BPH)	Likely
St. John's Wort	Depression	Likely
Yohimbe	Erectile dysfunction (ED), sexual dysfunction	Possibly

Other Common OTC Products

Condition or Symptom	Examples of Generic Names	Examples of Brand Names	Therapeutic Class
Acne	Benzoyl peroxide	Clearasil®, Acne Clear®, PanOxyl®	Topical acne remedy
	Salicylic acid	Clearasil®, Neutrogena®, Acne Clear®	Topical keratolyticskin exfoliant
Allergies (watery eyes, sneezing, itchy throat, runny nose)	Cetirizine	Zyrtec®	Antihistamine
	Chlorpheniramine	Chlor-Trimeton®, Zicam®	Antihistamine
	Clemastine	Tavist®	Antihistamine
	Cromolyn	NasalCrom®	Mast cell stabilizer
	Diphenhydramine	Benadryl®	Antihistamine
	Doxylamine	Unisom®, Nyquil Cold/Flu®, Zicam Max Strength Flu Nighttime®	Antihistamine
	Loratadine	Claritin®, Alavert®	Antihistamine
Cold sores/oral herpes	Docosanol	Abreva®	Antiviral agent
Constipation	Bisacodyl	Dulcolax®, Fleet®, Correctol®	Stimulant laxative
	Docusate sodium	Colase®, Dulcolax®	Emollient (stool softener)
	Glycerin (suppository)		Hyperosmotic laxative
	Magnesium citrate		Hyperosmotic laxative
	Magnesium hydroxide	Milk of Magnesia	Antacid and laxative
	Methylcellulose	Citrucel®	Bulk-forming laxative
	Mineral oil		Lubricant laxative
	Polycarbophil	FiberCon®	Bulk-forming laxative
	Psyllium hydrophobic mucilloid	Metamucil®	Bulk-forming laxative
	Sennosides	Ex-Lax®, Senna®	Stimulant laxative
Cough	Dextromethorphan	Delsym®, Hold DM®, Silphen DM®, Robitussin DM®, Diabetic Tussin®	Antitussive
	Guaifenesin	Mucinex®, Humibid®, Hytuss®, Robitussin®, Diabetic Tussin®	Expectorant
	Codeine	Robitussin A-C®, Cheracol®	Schedule V antitussive
Dandruff	Pyrithione zinc	Head and Shoulders®	Dandruff treatment
	Selenium sulfide	Head and Shoulders® Intensive Treatment	Dandruff treatment
Diaper rash	Zinc oxide	Destin®	Skin protectant

Condition or Symptom	Examples of Generic Names	Examples of Brand Names	Therapeutic Class
Diarrhea	Bismuth subsalicylate	Pepto-Bismol®, Kaopectate®	Antidiarrheal
	Loperamide	Imodium®	Antidiarrheal
Dry skin	Various ingredients: petrolatum, mineral oil, glycerin, propylene glycol, lecithin, dimethicone, urea, lactic acid, etc.	Lubriderm®, Eucerin®, Vaseline®, Curel®, LacHydrin®	Petrolatum, mineral oil, glycerin, propylene glycol, and lecithin = skin moisturizers. Dimethicone = skin protectant. Lactic acid and urea = exfoliants
Ear wax removal	Carbamide peroxide	Debrox®, Murine®, Otix®,	Wax-softening agent
Eye irritation (allergic conjunctivitis)	Carboxymethyl-cellulose	Clear Eyes® Lubricant for dry eyes	Lubricant
	Glycerin, hypromellose, and polyethylene glycol	Visine Tears®	Moisturizer
	Ketotifen	Alaway®, Zaditor®	Topical antihistamine
	Naphazoline	Clear Eyes Redness®, Visine-A®, Opcon-A®, Naphcon-A®	Topical decongestant
	Oxymetazoline	Visine L.R.®	Topical decongestant
	Pheniramine	Visine-A®, Opcon-A®, Naphcon-A®	Topical antihistamine
	Tetrahydrozoline	Clear Eyes Triple®, Visine Advanced®	Topical decongestant
Flatulence	Alpha-Galactosidase	Beano®	Digestive aid
	Simethicone	Gas-X®, Gas Relief®, Alamag Plus®	Antiflatulent
Fungal infections (ringworm, jock itch, athlete's foot, etc.)	Butenafine	Lotrimin Ultra®	Anti-fungal
	Clotrimazole	Lotrimin®	Anti-fungal
	Miconazole	Micatin®	Anti-fungal
	Terbinafine	Lamisil topical®	Anti-fungal
Headache, migraines, fever, or cramps	Acetaminophen (APAP)	Tylenol®, Children's Tylenol®	Analgesic
	Aspirin (ASA)	Bayer®, Bufferin®, St. Joseph®, Acuprin®	Analgesic
	APAP + ASA + Caffeine	Excedrin®	Analgesic
	Ibuprofen	Motrin®, Advil®, Midol®	Non-steroidal anti-inflammatory drug (NSAID)

Condition or Symptom	Examples of Generic Names	Examples of Brand Names	Therapeutic Class
	Naproxen	Aleve®	Non-steroidal anti-inflammatory drug (NSAID)
Heartburn/ GERD	Aluminum hydroxide	Mylanta®, Gaviscon®, Amphojel®, AlternGEL®, Basaljel®, Maalox®	Antacid
	Calcium carbonate	TUMS®, Maalox®, Rolaids®	Antacid
	Cimetidine	Tagamet®	H2-antagonist (anti-ulcer)
	Famotidine	Pepcid AC®	H2-antagonist (anti-ulcer)
	Magnesium hydroxide	Milk of Magnesia®, Rolaids®, Mylanta®, Mag-ox®, Ur-mag®, Gaviscon®, Maalox®	Antacid
	Nizatidine	Axid®	H2-antagonist (anti-ulcer)
	Omeprazole	Prilosec OTC®	Proton pump inhibitor (PPI) (anti-ulcer)
	Ranitidine	Zantac®	H2-antagonist (anti-ulcer)
	Sodium bicarbonate	Alka-seltzer®	Antacid
Hemorrhoids	Pramoxine	Preparation H®, Tronothane®, Tucks®	Topical anesthetic
Insomnia	Dipenhydramine	Benadryl®	Antihistamine
	Doxylamine	Unisom®, All-Nite®	Antihistamine
Itching (insect bites or stings, poison ivy, poison oak, etc.)	Benzocaine	Lanacane®, Sting-kill®	Topical anesthetic
	Benzyl alcohol	Itch-X®	Topical anesthetic
	Calamine	Aveeno Calamine®	Astringent skin protectant
	Hydrocortisone	Cortizone®, Cortaid®	Corticosteroid (anti-inflammarory agent)
	Lidocaine	Bactine®	Topical anesthetic
	Pramoxine	Itch-X®	Topical anesthetic
Lactose intolerance	Lactase enzyme	Lactaid®	Enzyme replacement
Lice	Lindane shampoo	Kwell Shampoo®, Scabene Shampoo®	Pediculocide

Condition or Symptom	Examples of Generic Names	Examples of Brand Names	Therapeutic Class
Minor skin cuts/ openings (antibiotics)	Isopropyl alcohol		Antiseptic
	Polymyxin B + Bacitracin	Polysporin®	Topical antibiotic
	Polymyxin B + Bacitracin + Neomycin	Neosporin®, Triple antibiotic	Topical antibiotic
Motion sickness	Dimenhydrinate	Dramamine®	Anti-nauseant
	Diphenhydramine	Benadryl®	Anti-nauseant
	Meclizine	Dramamine Less Drowsy®	Anti-nauseant
Nasal congestion (stuffy nose)	Levmetamfetamine	Vicks Vapor Inhaler®	Topical nasal decongestant
	Oxymetazoline	Afrin®	Topical nasal decongestant
	Pseudoephedrine*	Sudafed®, Drixoral®, Dimetapp®, Actifed®, Alavert®, Chlor-Trimenton®	Decongestant
	Phenylephrine	4-way®, Sudafed PE®, Neo-Synephrine®, Pediacare®	Topical nasal decongestant
Nausea and vomiting	Bismuth subsalicylate	Pepto-Bismol®, Kaopectate®	Antidiarrheal
	Phosphorated carbohydrate solution	Emetrol®	Antiemetic
Pain (back, arm, leg) (topical analgesics)	Benzocaine	Lanacane®, Sting-kill®	Topical anesthetic
	Capsaicin	Zostrix®	Counterirritant
	Lidocaine	Bactine®	Topical anesthetic
	Menthol	Bengay®, Thera-gesic®	Counterirritant
	Methyl salicylate	Icy Hot®, Thera-gesic®, WellPatch®, Flexall®	Counterirritant
	Trolamine salicylate	Aspercream®	Counterirritant
Sore throat	Benzocaine	Cepacol®, Halls®	Topical anesthetic
	Menthol	Cepacol®, Halls®	Topical antitussive
Smoking Cessation	Nicotine polacrilex	Nicorette gum®, Commit lozenge®, Nicoderm CQ® patch	Nicotine replacement therapy
Sunburn	Lidocaine with aloe	Solarcaine®	Topical anesthetic
Swimmer's ear	Isopropanol	Auro-Dri®, SwimEar®, StarOtic®	Ear drying agent
Warts	Salicylic acid	CompoundW®, DuoFilm®, Pedifix®	Exfoliant
Weight loss	Orlistat	Alli®	Lipase inhibitor

Pseudoephedrine must be kept behind the counter and has special requirements regarding the amount that may be purchased and the records that must be kept. In some states pseudoephedrine may be available only by prescription. Ask your pharmacist about the specific requirements for your state.

SELF-ASSESSMENT QUESTIONS
CHAPTER XIII

1. Pediculocides are used to:
    a. Treat athlete's foot.
    b. Kill lice.
    c. Treat itchy rashes.
    d. Treat insect bites.

2. Which of the following categories of OTC products can be used to treat constipation?
    a. Anti-flatulents.
    b. Decongestants
    c. Laxatives.
    d. Analgesics.

3. External analgesics can be used to:
    a. Treat athlete's foot.
    b. Clean wounds.
    c. Relieve the pain of hemorrhoids.
    d. Induce sleep.

4. Which of the following best describes a medication class used to treat bacterial infections?
    a. Antibiotic
    b. Antifungal
    c. Antiviral
    d. Antiseptic

5. Which of the following medications should be avoided by patients with high blood pressure?
    a. Sudafed
    b. Tylenol
    c. Benadryl
    d. Loratidine

Answers:
1) b
2) c
3) c
4) a
5) a

PHARMACY TECHNICIAN COMPETENCY ASSESSMENT
CHAPTER XIII

| Description of Ability or Skill | Initials | | Training Completed | |
	Tech	R.Ph.	Date	Remarks
The technician trainee can identify the major OTC categories and subcategories commonly found in a pharmacy.				
The technician trainee can describe the primary indication of major categories of OTC medications.				
The technician trainee can identify commonly used generic and brand-name OTC medications.				
The technician trainee can differentiate between the functions that may be performed by pharmacists versus pharmacy technicians with regard to OTC products.				
Identify common and severe adverse events that may occur when patients with certain conditions such as pregnancy, high blood pressure, diabetes, asthma, take contraindicated OTC medications.				
The technician trainee can describe major categories of vitamins and their primary indications.				

Chapter XIV
Unit Dose Systems and Drug Repackaging

Pharmacies that dispense prescriptions to patients residing in hospitals or long-term care facilities (LTCFs or nursing homes) may process prescription orders differently than the prescription processing system discussed in previous chapters of this *Training Program.* This chapter discusses these alternative drug distribution systems.

TYPES OF DRUG-DISTRIBUTION SYSTEMS

Although hospitals routinely use unit-dose distribution systems, pharmacists providing medications to patients in LTCFs may dispense them utilizing one of three types of drug-distribution systems:

- Traditional prescription vials
- Punch cards or blister packs
- Unit-dose packaging

Traditional Prescription Vials

Dispensing medications in prescription vials is time consuming for nurses working with LTCF patients. Using this system requires nurses to:

- Remove correct doses from labeled bottles
- Place medications in medicine cups lined up on a tray in the proper order
- Write medicine cards for each medication given stating:

    1.   Name of the patient
    2.   Name and strength of the medication dispensed
    3.   Times of administration

This method is the easiest one for the pharmacy, but requires a great deal of nursing time. It also creates more opportunities for medication errors.

Punch Cards or Blister Packs

The punch card or blister pack system consists of a cardboard card with rows of circular or oblong holes in it. Plastic bubbles or blisters stick out through these holes; each one holds one dose of medication. The back side of the bubble has a thin foil or paper backing through which the medication is pushed (or "punched"). This distribution system has several variations. For example, medications taken three times a day for 30 days are dispensed as 90 tablets or capsules in one card with three doses for each day of the month. A variation uses three separate 30-day cards—one each for morning, afternoon, and evening. Each card is labeled with the patient's name and bed number, the name of the medication, lot number and expiration date. A punch card system requires pharmacies to obtain a heat-sealing apparatus and movable carts for storage and administration of medications at the facility. The carts have removable cassettes to hold each patient's medications. The cassettes are exchanged at scheduled intervals

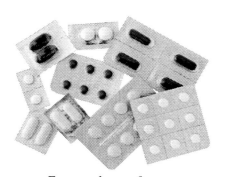

Examples of unit-dose packages

Unit-Dose Packaging

A unit-dose system dispenses medication in individually-packaged doses. The unit-dose container has the medication's name, lot number, and expiration date printed on its label. Some pharmaceutical manufacturers supply medications in prepackaged unit-dose containers. Other medications, particularly generics, are repackaged by pharmacies serving hospitals and LTCFs. Repackaging requires special equipment to fill and seal unit-dose containers. As with punch card systems, movable carts are used for storage and administration of medications at the facility.

There are several variations of unit-dose packaging including:

- 24-hour exchange
- 7-day exchange
- 15-day system
- 30-day system

The 24-hour and 7-day exchange systems or any variations require two sets of cassettes prepared identically. The nursing staff uses one set of cassettes while the other is at the pharmacy being refilled with medication. These cassettes are exchanged on a schedule. A 15-day or 30-day unit-dose system involves sending 15 or 30 days' supply of medication at one time.

Advantages of Punch Card and Unit-Dose Distribution Systems

While unused medications dispensed in prescription vials cannot be returned to the pharmacy, the environmentally-controlled and tamper-evident unit-dose packaging allows medications to be returned to the pharmacy for reuse in some states. Some states allow unused medications dispensed in punch cards to be returned to stock. The pharmacy can give credit to the payer for these unused doses. Another advantage of punch card and unit-dose packaging systems is that medication administration by nursing personnel is more efficient and accurate. This results in fewer medication errors and better recordkeeping. Although these systems cost more, their advantages are usually worth the extra cost. Long-term care facilities prefer these systems and some state Medicaid programs reimburse pharmacies more for prescriptions dispensed in unit-dose or punch card systems.

Note: Controlled substances must be locked in a secure place while they are stored at a LTCF. Medication carts have special locked compartments to accommodate these medications. Unused doses of controlled substances cannot be returned to the pharmacy for credit and are destroyed by a pharmacist.

Liquid medications can be sent to the LTCF in bulk containers (e.g., 4 oz or 16 oz bottles) or in unit-dose packaging. The bulk liquid medications are carried in the cart and can be poured just before they are administered to residents.

Each state governs correct prescription labeling for LTCFs. A pharmacist can describe your state's requirements.

While unit-dose repackaging offers several advantages, it also requires special procedures that you will have to follow carefully.

Practices for Repackaging

To protect medications' purity and potency, pharmaceutical manufacturers and pharmacies must meet specific guidelines when they package medications. Medication packaging takes four factors into consideration:

- **Identification.** Labels must describe the contents completely and precisely.

- **Protection from the environment.** Prescription containers must protect medications from the harmful effects of moisture, light, air, heat, and in the case of sterile products, from bacterial contamination.

- **Protection in handling.** Prescription containers must protect medication from breakage. The container itself must not interact chemically with the medication or allow medication to deteriorate.

- **Deliver the medication quickly, easily, and safely.** The package should not be an obstacle to getting to the medication.

Guidelines for Repackaging

When pre-packaged products are not available commercially, you may be assigned to repackage medications. Medications must be packaged according to your pharmacy department's established policies and procedures, and most importantly, according to the Commonwealth's repackaging regulations. Some general guidelines for repackaging medications are:

- Medication repackaging must be done in an isolated, clean area that allows enough space to work.

- Only one medication should be repackaged at a time. This reduces chances of confusing look-alike drugs or contaminating medications with residues from other medications.

- Before repackaging, check ingredients and labels carefully to verify that they are correct. Only labels for the medication currently being repackaged should be in the area; destroy unused labels for other medications immediately.

- Repackaged medications may not be released for distribution until checked and approved by a pharmacist.

- Repackaging equipment should be maintained according to manufacturers' instructions and cleaned after each repackaging operation. Records should be maintained on equipment maintenance, cleaning, and inspection.

- Keep complete and accurate records of each batch.

- Protect each dose from the environment during the repackaging process.

- Packaging materials used for prescription containers must be compatible with the medication.

- Label each dose with the medication's name, strength, lot number, and expiration date.

- Maintain written records for each batch for at least a year. (Some states require a longer time period.) These records should include:

  o The production date
  o Name of the medications repackaged
  o Lot numbers
  o Samples of labels
  o Description of containers
  o Equipment used
  o Initials of the pharmacist who checks the batch
  o Name of the person repackaging the medication

Expiration Dates on Repackaged Labels

Expiration dates assigned to repackaged medications ensure that products dispensed are effective at the time of use. Repackaging and exposing the medication to the environment may affect the medication's shelf life. Therefore, the expiration date you put on the label is not the same as the manufacturer's date. A pharmacist should determine the expiration date, but generally, the expiration date is the earlier of the following two choices:

1. The repackaged expiration date cannot be more than six months after the repackaging date; or

2. The repackaged expiration date cannot be more than 25 percent of the time between the original manufacturer's expiration date and the date of repackaging. For example, you repackage on August 31st and the expiration date on the manufacturer's original container is four months later, December 31st. The repackaged medication must show an expiration date no later than September 30, which is one month (25% of 4 months) after the repackaging date.

> **Note**: At the time of publication FDA was still currently considering a proposal to change the expiration dating for non-sterile, solid or liquid dosage forms repackaged in single-unit and unit-dose containers to the earlier of: (1) one year after the repackaging date or (2) the expiration date on the manufacturer's original container. Please check the "Manual Update" page on the ICPT website for any new information. http://www.nationaltechexam.org/tech_updates.shtml

EMERGENCY KITS

Hospitals and long-term care facilities have emergency kits (also known as "code carts" or "crash carts") that are used in emergency situations. These kits are used to store and organize emergency equipment and medication so that they are readily available when needed in an emergency. The kits are stored either as floor stock at nursing stations, in emergency rooms, in operating rooms or in a centralized pharmacy location. There are often separate emergency kits for newborn, pediatric and adult patients with the appropriate medications and supplies in each determined by hospital standard procedure.

Pharmacy technicians are often assigned the duty of checking these kits to determine whether any of the medications have been used and, if so, to make sure the medications are billed properly and restocked. Technicians may also be assigned the duty of checking expiration dates on all medications in the kit on a periodic basis and replacing expired or short-dated items. Each facility will have written policies and procedures for checking and restocking these kits. It is very important that the medications be stored in the correct area of the kit so that physicians and nurses can immediately find exactly what they need without searching. Please be sure to check with your pharmacist supervisor about your facility's policies and procedures.

COMPLIANCE AIDS

No matter how well pharmacists and pharmacy technicians prepare medications, their efforts are wasted if patients do not comply with their prescription directions.

Patient compliance can rise significantly when pharmacists counsel patients about the use of their medications and provide compliance aids. A "compliance aid" is anything that helps patients take the correct amount of medication at the correct time. Here are a few examples of compliance aids:

- **Dosage spoons.** Dosage spoons have hollow, tube-like handles, marked in milliliters (mL) and increments of one-fourth teaspoonful. The hollow handle measures the dose of medication and holds it to minimize spilling. Household teaspoons are inaccurate measuring devices for medication because their bowls are variously sized. Using dosage spoons increases the accuracy of the dose.

- **Cutter.** Useful for partial doses (such as one-half dose), the cutter's blades cleanly slice through the scored grooves on tablets to provide accurate doses.

Droppers. Droppers enable patients to accurately measure small quantities of liquid medications by either delivering medication one drop at a time or by filling the tube of the dropper up to a marked line on the tube.

- **Daily or weekly dose planner.** Handy compartmentalized containers are filled at the beginning of the day (or week) with the proper number of doses. The patient can then track how many doses have been taken for the day (or week). For example, the weekly dose planners contain compartments for each day, and then the day compartments are further subdivided into smaller compartments. Therefore, if a patient must take four tablets a day, all four sub-compartments for each day will contain a tablet. At the end of the day, the patient can verify that all compartments are empty.

- **Dial-a-dose dispenser.** The packaging resembles birth control packaging: as you dial the top plastic circle from day to day, a tablet or capsule is exposed or drops out of the container.

- **Flashing/beeping device.** These devices replace the caps on vials and operate on timers. They flash or beep at preset times, helping patients remember when to take their medication.

While compliance aids can be very helpful, they do have some potential problems. Medications are not always labeled properly and can be exposed to the harmful effects of air, moisture, or light. While pharmacists can dispense medications only in approved prescription containers (such as those described in the chapter entitled, "Prescription Medication"), they can help patients by showing them how to best use the various compliance aids.

Acknowledgment: Some information in this chapter was adapted with permission from Brown WM and Arnold JE, Long-Term Care Pharmacy: The Keys to Success in the '90s (Alexandria, VA: NARD, 1990):9-10.

1. Which of the following may sometimes be returned to the pharmacy for reuse in some states?
    a. Medication dispensed in traditional prescription vials.
    b. Medications dispensed in unit-dose packages.
    c. Controlled substances dispensed in punch cards
    d. None of the above may be returned for reuse.

2. If the manufacturer's label has an expiration date of December 31, 2009, and you repackage the medication into unit-dose containers on December 31, 2008, using USP-NF Class B packaging materials, the expiration date that you would put on the unit-dose package is:
    a. December 31, 2009.
    b. December 31, 2008.
    c. June 30, 2009.
    d. March 31, 2009.

3. When medications are repackaged into unit-dose containers, each dose must be labeled with the:
    a. Medication's name and strength
    b. Patient's name.
    c. Date the medication was repackaged in the unit-dose container.
    d. Name of the person responsible for repackaging

4. Which of the following is NOT a requirement for repackaging a medication?
    a The label must identify the contents completely and precisely.
    b The container must protect the medication from harmful effects of the environment.
    c The container must protect the medication from breaking.
    d The container must include some type of compliance aid.

5. According to the *Training Program,* written records for each batch of medication repackaged by a pharmacy should contain all the following information except:
    a The quantity prepared.
    b Date of repackaging.
    c Directions for use.
    d Name of the medication.

Answers:
1) b
2) d Note: The correct response will change if an FDA proposal goes into effect. See note in section on expiration dating.
3) a
4) d
5) c

PHARMACY TECHNICIAN COMPETENCY ASSESSMENT
CHAPTER XIV

| Description of Ability or Skill | Initials | | Training Completed | |
	Tech	R.Ph.	Date	Remarks
The technician trainee can explain the advantages and disadvantages of different types of drug-distribution systems (i.e., vials, punch cards and unit-dose packaging).				
The technician uses good practices for repackaging medications.				
The technician trainee can identify and explain the uses of compliance aids stocked in the pharmacy department.				

Chapter XV
Sterile Product Compounding

By: Kelly J. Burch
and Kenneth W. Schafermeyer

Note: New FDA regulations for preparing sterile products are expected to go into effect in June 2008. Any changes will be posted on the ICPT website at www.nationaltechexam.org under Updates. Please check the "Manual Update" page on the ICPT website for this new information.

STERILE DRUG PRODUCTS

As described in the chapter entitled, "Prescription Medication," drug products are delivered by many dosage forms and administration routes. This chapter focuses on drug products that are injected into the body through the skin. Another word used to describe these types of medications is "Parenteral," which literally means "outside the gastrointestinal tract." Although this word is used to describe any medication given by a route of administration other than oral or rectal, it is usually used to describe injectable medications.

Injectable drugs require special care and handling because they must be sterile. "Sterile" means that the product to be injected contains no bacteria (or germs) that could cause an infection. When sterile fluids are prepared, great care must be taken to avoid contaminating the product. Avoiding contamination (i.e., preventing the introduction of germs) is important because injected products bypass the body's natural defense systems, such as the skin and digestive tract, which are natural barriers to most germs. Because germs can multiply rapidly inside the body, it is extremely important to prevent contamination of injectable drugs so that patients do not get a serious infection.

Injectable drugs are used extensively in hospital pharmacies and almost every community pharmacy stocks some prepared and ready-to-use injectable products (such as insulin). Some injectable medications must be compounded in a pharmacy because dosages are customized for each patient (often according to the patient's body weight) and because some drugs are stable for only short periods of time after they are prepared (i.e., they have short shelf lives). To meet the specialized needs of these patients, pharmacies create the needed doses inside the pharmacy, using a process called "compounding."

Compounding sterile products requires special equipment and supplies. The process used to avoid contamination while compounding sterile products is known as "aseptic technique" and is described in detail later in this chapter. First, however, it is helpful to know more about the types of products, and the special supplies and equipment used in sterile compounding.

Types of Sterile Drug Products

In this *Training Program,* we classify sterile drug products three ways:
- Route of administration.
- Type of therapy.
- Volume of fluid.

Route of Administration. For injectable drugs there are three primary routes of administration:

- **Subcutaneous** (SubQ, SQ or SC) injections consist of very small volumes of fluid (usually less than one or two milliliters) given just below the skin using a fine, short needle. Insulin and allergy shots are common examples of subcutaneous injections. Patients often learn to give themselves SQ injections.

- **Intramuscular** (IM) injections also employ small volumes of fluid but are delivered deep into muscle tissue by longer and larger-bore needles. Because IM injections are more painful than SQ injections, they are usually administered by a physician or nurse. Sometimes an anesthetic medication, referred to as a "numbing" agent such as lidocaine, is given with an IM injection to make it less painful for the patient.

- **Intravenous (IV)** injections are delivered directly into the vein. The medication may be delivered all at once (i.e., an IV push) or slowly over a longer period of time, perhaps up to several hours or even days (i.e., a continuous infusion). For continuous infusion, a nurse places a flexible needle into an arm or hand vein for only two or three days allowing the medication container to be changed without removing the needle.

  Long-term IV therapy may require a more permanent IV placed by a surgeon. These types of IVs can last for months or years if the patient keeps the injection site clean and avoids getting an infection.

- **Intra-peritoneal** injections are particularly useful in laboratory animal medicine, in neonatal animals, and for the administration of large volumes. Absorption is via the portal system, which directs blood from the GI tract to the liver, so it is not useful for drugs that are removed by the liver. There is danger of infection, and peritoneal adhesions are not uncommon. These factors limit its use. Peritoneal dialysis is becoming more frequently used in small animals with short-term renal failure or insufficiency.

- **Intra-mammary** injections are useful when localized therapy is needed, for example in mastitis. It is important to remember that absorption into the systemic circulation may occur.

Type of Therapy. Among the types of parenteral drug therapy that may be delivered to outpatients are:

- **Total parenteral nutrition** (TPN) is used when patients cannot consume food or nutritional formula (like Ensure®) for a prolonged period of time. Each day, a carefully balanced solution containing sugar, protein, minerals, electrolytes, vitamins and water is administered to the patient. Some TPN patients require this treatment for a long time (years); others require it for a shorter period of time, for example, to improve their nutritional intake before or after an operation.

- **Antibiotics.** A patient with a resistant or chronic infection may need intravenous antibiotics for a long period of time. Once the correct antibiotic treatment is chosen for a particular infection, the patient may complete the treatment at home. The patient usually self-administers sterile antibiotic solutions on a set schedule.

- **Chemotherapy.** Cancer patients may receive chemotherapy at home. It is common for these patients to also receive other IV medications that help relieve some of the side effects of chemotherapy. Examples are antiemetic agents (to treat nausea and vomiting), colony stimulating factors (to increase the infection-fighting white blood cells) and IV fluids (to avoid dehydration).

- **Pain medication.** Some patients, particularly cancer patients, receive intravenous pain medications along with their other medications. With the use of a patient controlled analgesia (PCA) device, many patients regulate the frequency of administration of their own pain medication.

- **Other therapies** such as blood transfusions, immunoglobulins or injectable drugs for anemia are often prepared for hospital patients but may also be considered for home care. To be eligible for home care, the treatment must be for a predictable period of time and patients, or their caregivers, must have a basic understanding of their treatment and know the procedures that must be followed. Usually a nurse trains the patient or caregiver and checks on the patient periodically. A team of a doctor, nurse and pharmacist work with the patient and caregiver to determine whether home treatment is safe and desired.

Volume of Fluid. Sterile products are often classified according to volume.

- **Small-volume parenterals** contain just enough fluid volume to safely deliver the medication into a patient's vein. The fluid is less important than the drug product. These types of prescriptions are fairly easy to compound. An example of a prescription for a small volume parenteral is:

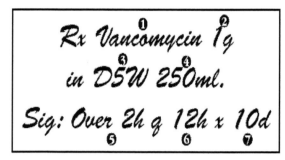

❶ Medication generic name
❷ Medication strength
❸ Diluent generic name ("D5W" = "Dextrose 5% in water")
❹ Diluent volume
❺ Infusion rate (infused over a 2-hour period)
❻ Frequency of administration (every 12 hours)
❼ Duration of therapy (for 10 days)

Prescription order for a small-volume parenteral

This prescription tells you to add one gram of vancomycin to a 250-mL container of dextrose 5% in water and give intravenously over a two-hour period, repeated every 12 hours for 10 days. ("D5W" is the abbreviation for dextrose 5% in water; other abbreviations can be found in Chapter IV of this *Training Program.)* Because of the relatively short shelf life of many IV medications, you would not prepare the entire twenty doses (10-day supply) at the same time. The pharmacist will consider a drug's stability when telling you how much to prepare.

When a small-volume parenteral is compounded, the correct drug, dose, dilution solution (called diluent) and number of doses all must be calculated and double checked prior to beginning the compounding process. Many small-volume parenterals are delivered into the vein at the same time as another fluid. They are said to be given "on piggyback" of the other fluid. An IV piggyback is a relatively small-volume medication that is usually administered along with a large-volume IV bag or preparation. The IV piggyback is put on top of the large-volume IV bag hence the term "piggyback." The products are usually mixed in the flexible tubing that is attached between the IV bags.

- **Large-volume parenterals** have a different purpose — they are used when the fluid itself is the treatment. This is the case with fluids used to prevent or treat dehydration. The most complicated type of large volume parenteral solution is total parenteral nutrition (TPN).

A prescription for a large-volume parenteral will specify the drug, amount of active ingredient, diluent, concentration and rate and duration of administration. For example, a chemotherapy patient might have the following prescription:

❶ ❷ *Rx: KCl 20 mEq* ❸ ❹ *in Dextrose 5%, half NS 1 L* *Sig: 75 ml/hr x3d* ❺ ❻	❶ Medication generic name ("KCl"= "Potassium Chloride") ❷ Medication strength (20 milliEquivalents) ❸ Diluent generic name (Dextrose 5% in water, half normal saline*) ❹ Diluent volume (one liter) ❺ Infusion rate (75ml per hour) ❻ Duration of therapy (for 3 days)

Prescription order for a large-volume parenteral

As you can see from the examples given, prescriptions for small-volume parenterals specify the frequency of administration; large-volume parenterals prescribe the rate of administration. Many large-volume solutions are manufactured to be used right off the shelf, with no additives needed. Others, known as "IV admixtures," may require the addition of one or more active ingredients. The fluids, any additives and the number to be compounded all must be checked carefully by both the technician and pharmacist before beginning any compounding. Most large-volume parenterals are relatively easy to compound. TPN solutions, however, require many steps and are probably some of the most difficult prescriptions to compound.

> **Note:** You must be very careful when preparing these products because the differences in product names are very subtle. For example, dextrose 5% and half normal saline sound a lot like dextrose 5% and quarter normal saline. The therapeutic difference between these solutions is great, so it is easy to see that pharmacists and technicians need to communicate carefully, and double check preparation of these prescriptions.

STERILE COMPOUNDING ENVIRONMENT

All parenteral medications must be sterile! The first step toward assuring product sterility is keeping the compounding area as clean as possible. However, circumstances do not always allow for every medication to be compounded within absolutely sterile environments; therefore, it is important to be aware of how to maintain as sterile a compounding environment as possible given a range of situations from least-to more-controlled environments.

The least-controlled environment is a countertop or table. Medications are sometimes compounded in this type of environment at the patient's bedside or home. The countertop must be clean (preferably wiped with isopropyl alcohol), the air must be relatively free of dust and the person doing the preparation must wash his or her hands very thoroughly. This method of compounding is usually not advised and can only be done when the product is used immediately so that bacteria inadvertently introduced into the product do not have time to multiply. Because of the risks involved, compounding on a countertop or table may not be appropriate for patients with weak immune systems (i.e., cancer or AIDS patients).

Laminar-Flow Hood

Medications for patients with weak immune systems and medications that are going to be stored for even a short period of time after preparation require a more controlled environment. A very important piece of equipment used to establish a sterile environment is a "laminar-flow hood" (or "hood" for short). The hood has a smooth non-porous surface, such as Formica or stainless steel, about the height and depth of a kitchen counter. At the back of the work surface, a grid holds a special filter with very small pore size — a "high efficiency particulate air" (HEPA) filter. The HEPA filter removes particles from the air. Although bacteria are smaller than the openings in the HEPA filter, most airborne bacteria are attached to particles floating in the air, so removing dust particles from the air removes the bacteria.

Virtually all pharmacies that compound sterile products have laminar-flow hoods. Most hospitals and some high-volume community pharmacies specializing in sterile product compounding have a special "clean room" to control the environment of the entire compounding area, not just the work surface where products are compounded. A room may contain more than one hood. There are two basic types of laminar-flow hoods: horizontal and vertical.

- Horizontal laminar-flow hood. As shown in the illustration, a horizontal laminar-flow hood has the filter perpendicular to the work surface. The clean air blows from the filter toward the person working in the hood, thereby keeping particulate matter away from the work surface. To maintain sterility, you must always keep your hands and any non-sterile materials or supplies "downwind" from the product.

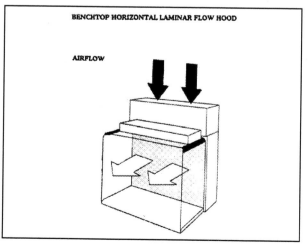

BENCHTOP HORIZONTAL LAMINAR FLOW HOOD

AIRFLOW

Reprinted with permission from the Policy and Procedure Manuals of New IV Therapeutics Corp., St. Louis, Missouri

While horizontal laminar-flow hoods are very effective and relatively inexpensive, they do have one disadvantage — they blow a mild current of air directly at the person doing the compounding, resulting in repeated contact with medications. Exposure to chemotherapy drugs and some antibiotics can cause serious problems and should be avoided by all personnel— especially women who are pregnant or nursing a child. It is recommended that these products be compounded in a vertical laminar-flow hood (also known as a "biological safety cabinet").

- Vertical laminar-flow hood. As shown in the accompanying illustration, a vertical hood's HEPA filter is parallel to the work surface and clean air blows straight down toward the work surface. The clean air is exhausted by a vent which surrounds the work surface. A glass or clear plastic screen on the front of the hood is pulled down so that hands can be inserted into the hood while the upper body and head are isolated from the air flow. The techniques for working safely and aseptically in a vertical hood are different than for a horizontal hood and, consequently requires different training.

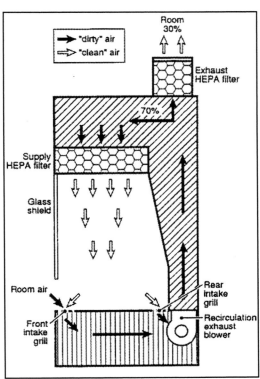

Class II, Type A
Biological Safety Cabinet

Maintaining a Sterile Compounding Environment

Because of the link between particles and bacteria, many of the operating procedures and rules about the compounding environment are directed at decreasing dust and dirt in the air near the hood. The hood should be located away from busy areas of the pharmacy department that have heavy foot traffic or, ideally, in a separate room built for sterile compounding only. Boxes and cartons create a lot of particulate matter and should not be stored near the compounding area. Many pharmacies have a policy of assembling all of the needed components of a prescription on a cart and spraying the cart and supplies with isopropyl alcohol before entering the compounding area. Computers and printers should not be near the hood. Pens, pencils, calculators and papers may be needed in the compounding area, but should not be in the hood. It goes without saying that food, drinks and cigarettes should never be in the compounding area.

Trash Disposal. Handling trash is an important but surprisingly complicated aspect of maintaining the compounding environment. The packaging of sterile products makes a lot of trash due to the protective packaging on supplies such as syringes and needles. Also, some of the products needing disposal require special handling. Syringes, needles, tubing and other supplies are packaged individually in protective paper and plastic to protect them from accidental contamination. This protective packaging can be disposed of in normal trash. Drug vials (other than those for chemotherapy drugs and some antibiotics) and empty containers for large-volume parenterals can usually be disposed of in normal trash. Check with the pharmacist about your policy on trash disposal.

Biomedical Waste Disposal. Any materials that may come into contact with chemotherapy drugs and certain antibiotics should be regarded as biomedical waste and must be disposed of separately for environmental reasons. "Sharps," such as used needles or broken glass, are also regarded as biomedical waste and are usually disposed of in a plastic box that is designed to prevent materials from being retrieved once they have been discarded. Chemotherapy products and "sharps" may require handling different than non-chemotherapy products and "sharps." Therefore, biomedical containers containing chemotherapy products and "sharps" may be labeled differently from non-chemotherapy biomedical containers. Check with the pharmacist about biomedical waste disposal. Biomedical waste is discarded separately and usually incinerated. Since disposal of biomedical waste is expensive, it is important to put only biomedical waste in the containers designated for this purpose.

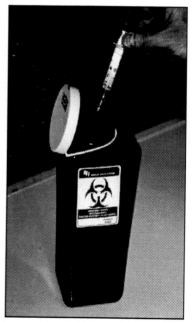

Biomedical Waste Container

Patient Records Disposal. A final aspect of waste disposal concerns records that could identify patients. When office paperwork is discarded, it is best to shred any document that could contain sensitive patient information. Of course, this shredding should not be done near the sterile compounding area.

Using Aseptic Techniques

To maintain a sterile environment, pharmacists and pharmacy technicians must learn to use "aseptic technique"— a series of steps and precautions that are used to decrease the chance of contamination during preparation of a sterile product.

Personal preparations. First, prepare yourself to enter the compounding area by removing all jewelry (including rings, watches and bracelets) and wash your hands thoroughly with warm water and antibacterial soap. Many pharmacies recommend or require that pharmacists and technicians do not wear cosmetics or nail polish when compounding sterile products. Some pharmacists and technicians use a special alcohol foam after properly washing their hands with antibacterial soap and water.

> **Note:** Remember that every time you have to handle objects outside of the hood, you must wash your hands again before putting them back in the sterile environment of the hood.

Some pharmacies require additional precautions. Be sure to check with the pharmacist to determine whether the following are required:
- Cover gowns
- Disposable hair covers
- Disposable facemasks
- Disposable shoe covers
- Disposable gloves

> **Note:** While these precautions decrease the particles in the compounding area and may be helpful, none of these precautions substitute for good hand washing. Many pharmacies require pharmacists and technicians to wash protective gloves with an alcohol solution after they are put on.

Hood work surface preparation. Before beginning the compounding procedure, disinfect the work surface of the hood by pouring a small amount of alcohol in a line at the back of the work surface and wiping with a sterile lint-free pad. To avoid contaminating the cleanest part of the work surface with particles from the dirtier parts, be sure to wipe from the filter to the front edge of the work surface in a broad side-to-side motion. (Instead of pouring a small amount of alcohol onto the work surface, you may use a spray bottle of alcohol instead, but be sure you do not spray alcohol directly into the filter.)

Compounding Procedures. The actual aseptic compounding procedures vary depending upon the type of product compounded. Since pharmacies can use different types of equipment and supplies, it is possible that the procedures used in your pharmacy vary slightly.

Most aseptic compounding procedures involve two basic operations:
1. Withdrawing fluid from a container and
2. Transferring it to another container.

Because small amounts must be measured carefully in an aseptic environment, sterile needles and syringes are used to transfer fluid from one container to another. While this sounds simple, it takes practice to do this accurately while maintaining sterility.

Air is cleanest near the HEPA filter. At the edge of the work surface, the air is barely different from the outside environment, so it is important to keep the product you are using at least six inches inside the edge of the hood. The product should be bathed in the flow of the cleanest possible air so other bottles, your hands or any other potential source of contamination should not be between the clean product and the clean air filter. The non-porous surface should be cleaned frequently with an antibacterial liquid, such as isopropyl alcohol. Trash should be removed often. Each pharmacy has specific procedures for these maintenance jobs. A log is usually maintained to document that these important tasks are carried out regularly.

Following are standard procedures used for some of the most common types of products. The pharmacist should tell you if the pharmacy's procedures vary from these. The first step is to withdraw fluid from either a multiple-dose vial or an ampule.

Components of a syringe

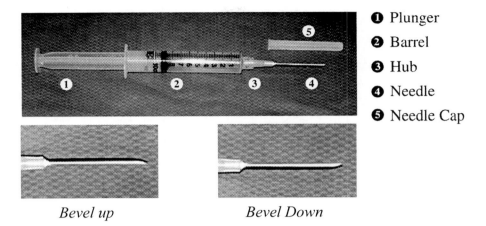

❶ Plunger
❷ Barrel
❸ Hub
❹ Needle
❺ Needle Cap

Bevel up   *Bevel Down*

Procedure for withdrawing fluid from a multiple-dose vial:

1. Choose the correct syringe size.
2. Remove the syringe from its package.
3. Remove the plastic cap from the tip of the syringe, without touching the tip.
4. Either lay the syringe on the work surface in the laminar-flow hood, without touching the tip to the work surface, or stand it up, using the top of the plunger as a stand.
5. Choose the appropriate size needle.
6. Remove the packaging from the needle, without touching the hub.
7. Screw the needle onto the tip of the syringe (usually about a quarter turn will adequately join the two).
8. Pull the cap straight off the needle.
9. Remove the protective plastic cap off the vial and use an alcohol swab to clean the rubber port on the top of the vial.
10. Pull back the plunger of the syringe to the desired volume that you want to extract. Do not touch any portion of the syringe plunger.
11. Place the bevel of the needle facing up, on top of the vial closure.
12. Push the needle into the vial at a 45 degree angle with the bevel facing up to prevent coring*.
13. Inject the air from the syringe into the container.

Note: If you are withdrawing from a flexible plastic container, you may skip the steps of injecting air. These are important steps in withdrawing from a glass container but can be omitted if the container will collapse as fluid is withdrawn.

---

*Coring is a condition where a core or hole is made in the rubber covering the vial. Coring is bad because it increases the risk of contaminating the medication. Coring can also plug the needle, which can make it difficult to draw the medication into the syringe.

Removing fluid from a multiple-dose vial. Air is injected into the vial before the medication is drawn into the syringe Hands should never be between the HEPA filter and the medication.

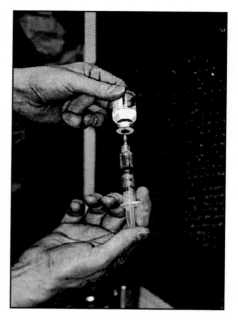

14. Allow the air pressure in the vial to help you withdraw the desired amount of fluid.
15. Hold the syringe with the needle straight up (like a rocket) to allow air bubbles to collect at the top of the syringe.
16. Push the air bubbles back into the vial and recheck to verify that the syringe has the correct amount of fluid.
17. Withdraw the needle. If you need to put this filled syringe down, either lay it carefully on the work surface (without touching the needle to the work surface) or stand it up, using the top of the plunger as a stand. Avoid recapping the needle.

Procedure for reconstituting powdered medication in a vial. Some vials are supplied as powders that must be reconstituted (i.e., the powder, must be dissolved in a liquid just before use). In this case, the following steps must be taken:

1-17. Complete steps 1-17 as described on the previous two pages.
18. Withdraw the correct amount of fluid to dissolve the powder, referred to as a diluent, from a multiple-dose vial or plastic container.
19. Remove the plastic protective cap off the vial containing the powder to be reconstituted and use an alcohol swab to clean the rubber port on the top of the vial.
20. Place the needle bevel up on the vial and insert the needle.
21. Inject the diluent into the vial. (You may have to do this a little at a time, allowing air to bubble into the syringe if needed.)
22. Withdraw the needle and discard.
23. Make sure the powder is dissolved — you may have to shake the vial carefully.
24. After the powder is dissolved, withdraw the appropriate amount of fluid from the vial using the procedure described for withdrawing fluid from a multiple-dose vial. To add the fluid to a piggyback or large-volume parenteral, refer to the procedure that follows later in this chapter.

Procedure for withdrawing fluid from an ampule. An ampule is a special type of glass container that does not have a rubber closure. To open and measure the fluid in an ampule, follow the following steps:

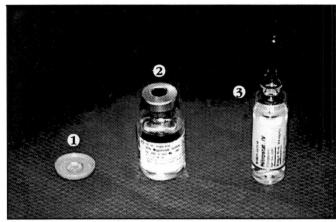

Examples of a 10mL multiple-dose vial (left) and a 10mL ampule (right)

❶ *Plastic cap removed from vial*

❷ *Rubber injection port at top of vial*

❸ *Neck where ampule is broken to open*

1-8. Assemble the needle and syringe as described in steps 1-8 above.
9. Using an alcohol swab clean the neck of the ampule.
10. Tap the ampule on the work surface to assure that all the fluid is in the bottom of the container.
11. Wrap an alcohol wipe or sterile gauze around the neck of the ampule.
12. Place thumbs against ampule neck and break away from yourself and the HEPA filter. Discard the top.
13. Insert the tip of the needle into the fluid and pull back on the syringe.
14. Tip the ampule if needed to remove the desired amount of fluid.
15. Replace the plastic cap on the needle.
16. Change the needle on the syringe to a filter needle to filter any small glass particles from the fluid as it is added to the final product.

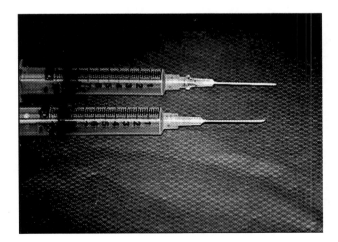

Syringe with filter needle (top) and syringe with standard needle.

Procedure for adding fluid to a piggyback or large-volume parenteral. Once the correct amount of fluid has been withdrawn and measured, you will be adding it to another container.

1. Place the piggyback or LVP in the hood with the additive port nearest the HEPA filter.
2. Use an alcohol swab to clean the additive port.
3. Insert the needle straight into the additive port, but be careful not to puncture the sides of the injection port and be sure to choose a needle long enough to puncture the inner seal at the injection port (longer than 1/2 inch).
4. Inject the fluid into the container.
5. Withdraw the needle.
6. Invert the container several times to assure adequate mixing. The container should be visually inspected against a white and black background for particulate matter and leakage.

DISPENSING STERILE PRODUCT PRESCRIPTIONS

The process of dispensing sterile products includes some steps before and after the actual compounding procedures. The first step is for the pharmacist to receive the prescription and to prepare the compounding instructions for the technician. The physician prescribed the medication and the pharmacist will decide how many doses to compound, how much fluid and what fluids should be used and what package sizes of drugs should be used. The pharmacist will consider the stability of the drug, the clinical status of the patient and practical considerations such as how often medication will be administered to the patient. The pharmacist and nurse, considering the patient's needs, collaborate to decide whether the medication will be delivered intravenously by gravity flow or by pump (and if the latter, which type of pump). The pharmacist and nurse also decide on the types of tubing, filters and other IV supplies will be needed. Once these decisions are made, the pharmacist will record these decisions and will prepare the labels.

You and the pharmacist will need to discuss the compounding technique for the prescriptions. At first, this will require much discussion and supervision, but eventually, you will become more familiar with the supplies needed and the techniques used. You may want to make a list of all drugs, solutions, diluents, labels and containers needed. Check the compounding area to make sure that all the supplies needed are there; if not, gather them as you assemble the remaining components of the prescription. The pharmacist may want to check to make sure you have everything before you begin to compound. It is helpful to visualize or talk through the compounding process while you are doing your hand washing. This is a good double check of your supplies and fluids, and helps you plan your work. Once you have entered the compounding area, try to avoid answering the telephone or using a calculator or reference materials, since these things are likely to be dirty. That is why thinking through the compounding process before beginning is a valuable habit to develop. If you are called away from the procedure before you finish, try to leave a visual reminder of what is finished or make a note. If you are interrupted and have touched any objects outside the hood, be sure to wash your hands again prior to resuming the compounding process.

After you finish preparing a batch of products, the pharmacist will perform a final check of your work. To allow an accurate assessment of your work, leave out all empty containers and syringes with the plungers pulled back to show the volumes of the medications that you used. While the pharmacist is checking your work, you can clean up any spills in the hood using sterile lint-free pads.

The compounded medication is only one part of preparing sterile products; you may be expected to select the proper tubing, pumps, filters, syringes, needles and other IV supplies needed by the patient. It is important that you supply the correct materials in the right quantities. The pharmacist will double check not only the compounded medication, but also the IV supplies that are to be delivered with the medication.

Documentation

Sterile compounding requires a great deal of record keeping to satisfy the patient care and business needs of the pharmacy department. Documentation and record keeping provide information that is directly applicable to the formulation being compounded, a basis for the professional judgment and legal liability and they provide for consistency when formulations are compounded

- **Compounding process.** Each step of the compounding process is documented to verify that the proper procedures were used. There may be a variety of procedures for the different sterile products compounded within your pharmacy. For example, the American Society of Health-System Pharmacists classifies sterile products according to risk levels, ranging from Level I (least) to Level III (greatest) potential risk referring to the quality of the product. Some factors used to determine the risk level of a sterile product include storage conditions, complex compounding procedures, patients with weak immune systems and time between compounding and use by the patient. The pharmacist is responsible for assigning a risk level to a specific sterile product. Check with the pharmacist and become familiar with your pharmacy's compounding procedures.

- **Materials used.** The materials needed to compound each prescription are care-fully counted and recorded. This is done partly in order to avoid medication and compounding errors and partly to prepare an accurate bill. All other supplies are counted and a record is kept of what is delivered to the patient.

- **Controlled substances.** Controlled substance records are kept in a perpetual inventory, complicated by the fact that partial containers of sterile products may have limited storage life or must be both refrigerated and secured.

- **Inventory records.** Purchasing records, want books and receiving records are similar to more traditional practice, although you are likely to be surprised by the high costs of some home infusion drugs.

- **Clean room maintenance.** Records of clean room maintenance are kept, including frequent hood cleaning and less frequent pre-filter changes and hood certification inspections.

- **Quality assurance and quality control.** When compounding sterile products, assuring the sterility of the product and keeping the compounding area clean are essential. To achieve these objectives, sterile product compounding and equipment must be handled according to your pharmacy's established policies and procedures for quality assurance and quality control of sterile products, equipment and the environment. Check with the pharmacist and become familiar with your pharmacy's quality assurance and quality control policies and procedures.

- **Patient records.** Pharmacies keep additional records of each communication with patients, nurses, physicians, laboratories and insurance providers. Instead of filing prescriptions by number, you are likely to file all documents related to one patient together in that patient's file or chart.

Labeling

Once the prescription is prepared, each dose must be labeled. Usually the pharmacist will check the products that you compound before they are labeled. During the short time while finished products are not labeled, it is critical that all drug vials and other products be kept together with the labels. Unlabeled products are easy to misidentify and can be very dangerous. Carts or bins are usually used to help keep things organized.

After the pharmacist checks your work, you may be asked to help apply the labels to the medication containers. In most states, all legend drug containers must be labeled, including saline and heparin solutions used for flushing IV lines. Try to prevent the pharmacy label from obscuring any information preprinted on any medicine containers. Most patients and caregivers appreciate it when all doses are labeled with the labels facing the same way.

Labels for sterile products usually contain the following. The exact format of the label, as illustrated below, will vary from pharmacy to pharmacy.

- Hospital or pharmacy name, address and telephone number
- Patient name
- Prescription date
- Prescriber name
- Compounding date
- Medication/additive name and strength
- Diluent name and volume
- Final volume
- Sig/directions
- Administration instructions (frequency, rate and duration of infusion)
- Date and time for administration of medication
- Pharmacist identification
- Technician identification
- Expiration date and time

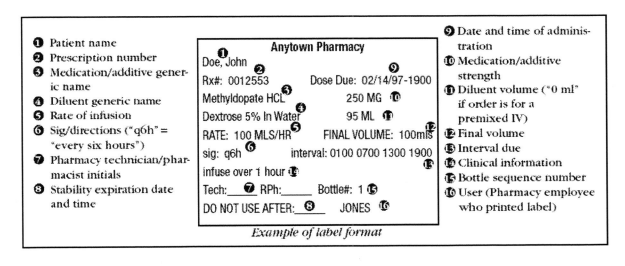

❶ Patient name
❷ Prescription number
❸ Medication/additive generic name
❹ Diluent generic name
❺ Rate of infusion
❻ Sig/directions ("q6h" = "every six hours")
❼ Pharmacy technician/pharmacist initials
❽ Stability expiration date and time

Anytown Pharmacy
Doe, John ❶
Rx#: 0012553 ❷   Dose Due: 02/14/97-1900 ❾
Methyldopate HCL ❸   250 MG ❿
Dextrose 5% In Water ❹   95 ML ⓫
RATE: 100 MLS/HR ❺   FINAL VOLUME: 100mls ⓬
sig: q6h ❻   interval: 0100 0700 1300 1900 ⓭
infuse over 1 hour ⓮
Tech:____ ❼ RPh:____   Bottle#: 1 ⓯
DO NOT USE AFTER:____ ❽   JONES ⓰

Example of label format

❾ Date and time of administration
❿ Medication/additive strength
⓫ Diluent volume ("0 ml" if order is for a premixed IV)
⓬ Final volume
⓭ Interval due
⓮ Clinical information
⓯ Bottle sequence number
⓰ User (Pharmacy employee who printed label)

COMPOUNDING EQUIPMENT AND SUPPLIES

Many types of compounding equipment may be needed for sterile product compounding. The following is a description of some of the more common equipment that you may encounter.

- If a large volume of fluid needs to be accurately measured and transferred to another container, a pump may be used.
- An automated compounder may be used in TPN compounding. This device combines a pump with an accurate balance. A computer interface can allow the pharmacist to direct the device to measure specific volumes of each additive, while also completing quality control and prescription documents.
- A repeater pump can ease the job of filling many small volume parenterals.
- A heat sealer or hand crimping tool may be needed to close bags of TPN solutions or other large-volume fluids.

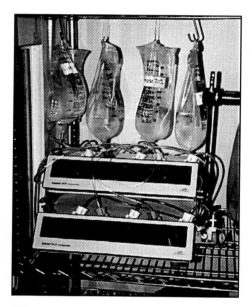

Clintec Automix 3+3 Compounder for preparing TPN solutions

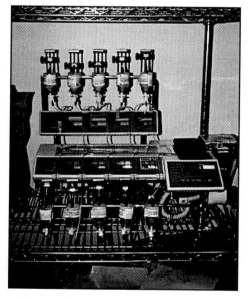

Clintec Micromix for adding small volumes of minerals to TPN

You will be oriented to needed equipment and supplies. You will be trained to operate some types of equipment. You will maintain other equipment so that the pharmacist has the necessary supplies ready to use.

Often some type of disposable supplies or tubing are needed to make equipment work correctly, and it may be your responsibility to stock the supplies or set up the machine and tubing. The pharmacist checks your work to assure that the correct set up is in place and the machine is programmed correctly, usually before you begin the compounding process.

SELF-ASSESSMENT QUESTIONS CHAPTER XV

1. Administration of medication into a patient's vein all at once (rather than over several hours or days) is known as a(n):
   a. SubQ injection.
   b. IM injection.
   c. IV push
   d. Continuous infusion.

2. Filter needles are used when:
   a. Reconstituting powdered medication in a vial.
   b. A laminar-flow hood is not available and medication must be compounded on a tabletop.
   c. The mediation being compounded is not sterile.
   d. Medication from an ampule is used.

3. A TPN is a type of:
   a. IM injection.
   b. SQ injection.
   c. Large-volume parenteral.
   d. Small-volume parenteral.

4. Labels prepared by the pharmacy for sterile products include all of the following except:
   a. Diluent name and volume.
   b. Stability expiration date and time.
   c. Date and time medication is to be administered.
   d. All of the above are included on the label.

5. Small-volume parenterals are:
   a. Designed to prevent the patient from dehydrating.
   b. Designed to provide the patient's nutritional needs.
   c. Often delivered as "piggybacks" along with large volume fluids.
   d. Generally used to specify the rate of administration.

Answers:
1) c
2) d
3) c
4) d
5) c

PHARMACY TECHNICIAN COMPETENCY ASSESSMENT
CHAPTER XV

Description of Ability or Skill	Initials		Training Completed	
	Tech	R.Ph.	Date	Remarks
The technician trainee can explain why parenteral drugs must be sterile.				
The technician trainee can identify and differentiate routes of administration for parenteral drugs.				
The technician trainee can give examples of the types of therapy that use parenteral drugs.				
The technician trainee uses proper aseptic technique.				
The technician trainee documents and labels parenteral prescriptions according to state regulations.				

Glossary

Active Ingredient - A small quantity of chemicals which produces a desired effect in the body. Active ingredients are combined with inactive ingredients to make convenient dosage forms.

Aerosol - Sprayable product most commonly used for topical application to the skin or for inhalation into the lungs and nasal passages.

Anesthetic Creams and Ointments - Medications used for treating irritating and itchy rashes, insect bites, stings, and sunburns.

Antacid- Medication used to reduce stomach acid; useful in treating heartburn or upset stomach.

Antibiotic- A substance derived from a mold, bacterium, or synthetic process that inhibits the growth of other microorganisms.

Anti-diarrheal - Medication used to reduce or stop diarrhea

Antiflatulent- Medication used to reduce discomfort of gas in stomach or intestines.

Applicator Bottle - A container that has a slender, glass or plastic rod attached to the inside of its cap. The rod has a bulb-like end which acts as an applicator for liquids.

Antiemetic - A substance which prevents or stops vomiting.

Aseptic Technique - A series of steps and precautions that are used to decrease the chance of contamination during preparation of a sterile product.

Assignment of Claims - Common provision in a participating pharmacy agreement that specifies that the pharmacy, rather than the patient, will send claims to a third-party payer.

Auxiliary Label - Supplemental label, other than the prescription label, that conveys instructions to the patient.

Average Wholesale Price (AWP) - The published "list price" of a particular drug product. Most pharmacies are able to purchase at discounts below AWP.

Bay- Storage area that is usually a U-shaped shelving unit in which medications are kept.

Blood Glucose Meter- Device used to measure the concentration of sugar in the blood. People with diabetes use this device to measure their blood sugar levels.

Brand Name - The trademark name given to products by their manufacturers.

Buccal Tablet - Tablet that is placed in the buccal pouch (i.e., the area between the cheek and gums) to allow the active ingredients to be absorbed directly into the blood stream.

Capitation Fee - A form of reimbursement in which a pharmacy is paid a specified amount of money each month for each patient who is assigned to receive prescriptions from that pharmacy. The pharmacy keeps the capitation payment for a particular patient whether or not that patient actually receives a prescription during that month. However, the pharmacy is obligated to dispense to that patient all prescriptions that the patient needs for that month even if the cost exceeds the monthly capitation fee payment.

Capsule - A small, oblong gelatin container filled with medication.

Claims Reconciliation - The process of comparing claims submissions to claims payments to detect incorrect claims rejections, as well as underpayments or overpayments.

Closed Panel - A network of pharmacies organized by a MCO or PBM in which only selected or preferred pharmacies may participate. These preferred pharmacies are often selected because they belong to a chain that is willing to accept lower reimbursement or share some of the MCO's administrative costs.

Coinsurance - A form of patient cost sharing in which patients pay a specified percentage of their medical expenses.

Collodion - Liquid medication that dries as a flexible film on the skin. Many wart, corn and callous remedies are prepared as collodions.

Compliance Aid - A device or system that helps remind patients to take the correct amount of medication at the correct time.

Compounding - Combining active and inactive ingredients to form a pharmaceutical product, sterile or non-sterile, that is not commercially available.

Continuous Infusion - A type of administration of intravenous medication in which a flexible needle is placed into a vein for only two or three days allowing the medication container to be changed without removing the needle. Long-term IV needle therapy may require a more permanent IV placed by a surgeon.

Contraindication - A symptom or medical condition which indicates the inappropriateness of a form of treatment that would otherwise be advisable.

Controlled-Release Product - A tablet, capsule or medication particles with special coatings designed to release the medication in the body a constant rate.

Controlled Substance - Drug with the potential for abuse or physical and/or psychological dependence.

Convalescent Aids - Medical devices such as canes, crutches, bed pans, cervical collars, etc.

Copayment - A form of patient cost sharing in which patients pay a fixed amount each time a prescription is dispensed.

Covered entity - an entity that is a health care provider that conducts certain transactions in electronic form, a healthcare clearinghouse, and/or a health plan.

Cream - Preparation combining water, oil and other substances. Although they usually do not offer as much protection as ointments, creams are more appealing to patients because they are absorbed by the skin and usually are not greasy or oily.

Days Supply - The number of days that a prescription should last if a patient takes the medication according to directions.

DDS, DMD - Dentist.

DEA Number - A number assigned to a prescriber which documents his or her authority to prescribe controlled substances. Each pharmacy is also assigned a DEA number which documents its authority to stock and dispense controlled substances.

Deductible - A form of patient cost sharing. The amount that must be incurred and paid by the patient during a specified period of time before benefits are paid by the insurance company.

Disclosure - all pertinent information necessary for an informed decision is made available to a patient.

Dispense as Written (DAW) - A request by a prescriber that a pharmacist dispense the brand-name medication prescribed rather than a generic equivalent. Some third parties will reimburse pharmacies for multiple-source brand-name medications when prescribers insist on brand names.

Dispensing Fee - The portion of the third-party prescription reimbursement that is paid in addition to reimbursement for drug costs. This fee is supposed to cover the pharmacy's overhead and profit. Usually this is a fixed fee, meaning it is the same for every prescription dispensed.

DO - Osteopath.

DPM - Podiatrist.

Dropper Bottle - A bottle designed to deliver a very small volume of medication at a time. These bottles may have droppers attached to the inside of their caps or may have small openings that allow administration of one drop of medication at a time.

Drug Enforcement Administration (DEA) - Federal agency that regulates manufacturing, distribution, prescribing, and dispensing of controlled substances.

Drug-Disease Alert Procedure - A procedure that is followed when the pharmacy computer system identifies a potential drug therapy problem such as a contraindication, drug interaction, or non-compliance.

Drug Interaction - A situation in which the effect of one medication is changed by another medication that a patient is taking at the same time. These "Drug interactions" are usually classified in computer systems by their severity.

Drug Utilization Review - A process in which patterns of prescribing, dispensing and usage of prescription drugs are monitored. DUR may be prospective or retrospective.

Durable Medical Equipment - "Durable" or long-lasting medical devices or patient aids such as wheelchairs, walkers, or hospital beds.

DVM - Veterinarian.

Effervescent Tablet - A medication dosage form containing mixtures of acids and sodium bicarbonate, plus active ingredients, that is dissolved in a glass of water which the patient drinks.

Electronic Claims Adjudication - The process of using a computer and modem to determine whether a third-party claim will be paid, and if so, the amount of payment the pharmacy can expect to receive.

Elixir - Clear hydroalcoholic liquid intended for oral use, often containing flavoring agents.

Emulsion - Oil and water mixture which, in time, usually separates into an oil layer on top and a water layer on the bottom. Emulsions must be shaken before use.

Enteric-Coated Tablet - Tablet with a coating designed to allow it to pass through the stomach intact so that it dissolves in the intestine instead.

Enzyme - Medication that aids in digestion or reduces nausea.

Facing the Stock Bottles - Pulling merchandise forward to the edge of the shelf when restocking inventory.

Federal Upper Limit (FUL) - A list of multiple-source medications and their upper limits for state Medicaid program reimbursement.

Fee-for-Service - Traditional indemnity type of business insurance that provides coverage for health care services to members. With this type of coverage, providers are paid a fee for each service delivered, in contrast to capitated systems in which a fixed amount is paid in advance for all services that may be provided during a given period of time (usually a month).

Fluid Extract or Tincture - Medication dosage form in which the active ingredients (often a plant extract) is dissolved in a base of alcohol and/or water.

Food and Drug Administration (FDA) - The federal agency that supervises the development, testing, purity, safety, and effectiveness of prescription and OTC medications.

Formulary - A list of medications that are covered (or not covered) by a third-party prescription program.

Gel - Semisolid suspension of very small particles, usually in a water base.

Generic Drug - Multiple-source drug that does not have a brand name. Also known as a "generic equivalent."

Generic Name - The official or chemical name of a product's active ingredients.

Generic Substitution - A process of substituting the lower-cost generic version of a medication when a brand-name medication is prescribed. Generic substitution is often mandated by third-party payers to reduce prescription costs.

Health Maintenance Organization (HMO) - A type of third-party plan in which providers share risks with the insurance company by being obligated to provide health care services in return for a fixed amount of reimbursement for each patient assigned to them. Patients are often required to use only those health care providers to whom they are assigned.

High-Efficiency Particulate Air (HEPA) Filter - A special filter used in laminar-flow hoods that is designed to remove small particles and bacteria from the air.

Hydroalcoholic - Those liquids that contain a combination of alcohol and water.

Incidental disclosure - personal information is shared unintentionally with unauthorized users during the performance of daily operations.

Indemnification - A reimbursement mechanism in which the patient pays the pharmacy and is later reimbursed by the insurance company for a portion of the cost. (Note the difference between indemnification and assignment of claims.)

Intramuscular (IM) - Injections employing small volumes of fluid that are delivered deep into muscle tissue by relatively longer and larger-bore needles.

Intravenous (IV) - Injectable medication that is administered intravenously (into the vein).

IV Push - Medications given intravenously over a short period of time.

Laminar-Flow Hood (Horizontal) - A horizontal laminar-flow hood has the HEPA filter perpendicular to the work surface. The clean air blows from the filter toward the person working in the hood, thereby keeping particulate matter away from the work surface.

Laminar-Flow Hood (Vertical) - A vertical laminar-flow hood's HEPA filter is parallel to the work surface and clean air blows straight down toward the work surface. A glass or clear plastic screen on the front of the hood is pulled down so that hands can be inserted into the hood while the upper body and head are isolated from the air flow. The techniques for working safely and aseptically in a vertical hood are different than for a horizontal hood.

Laxative - Medication used to relieve constipation, rectify incomplete or irregular bowel movements, or evacuate the bowel.

Legend Statement - Medications that can be dispensed only by prescription have either a "Rx-only" symbol or the following statement (or legend) on their labels: "Caution: Federal law prohibits dispensing without prescription." For this reason, prescription-only medications are also known as "legend drugs."

Liniment - Mixture of various substances in oil, alcoholic solutions of soap, or emulsions intended for external application; often used for their heat-producing effects.

Long-Term Care Facility (LTCF) - Facility where patients reside and are cared for by trained personnel for an extended time period. Also referred to as a "nursing home" or a "skilled nursing facility."

Lotion – Although similar to a cream, this medication dosage form contains more liquid and is applied more easily over larger areas of the body.

Lot Number - A number that identifies medications as belonging to particular batches produced by the manufacturer. It is sometimes called a "control number."

Maintenance Medication - Pharmaceutical used to treat or manage chronic long-term conditions and illnesses.

Managed Care Organization (MCO) - An organization designed to manage the cost and quality of and access to health care services.

Maximum Allowable Cost (MAC) - The maximum amount that will be paid by a third-party payer for a multiple-source medication. For example, a third-party payer sets the MAC at the level of a lower-cost generic equivalent that is readily available from wholesalers and reimburses pharmacies at this level whether a brand-name medication or its generic equivalent is dispensed.

MD - Physician, usually an allopathic physician (as opposed to an osteopathic physician).

Meniscus - The surface of a liquid in which surface tension causes the liquid to cling to the sides of a container. When measuring liquids in a graduated cylinder, one should measure from the bottom of the meniscus.

Multiple-Source Drug - A drug product that is available from more than one manufacturer.

NDC Number - The national drug code (NDC) is assigned by the manufacturer and placed on all prescription stock packages. The NDC number identifies the manufacturer, the actual chemical entity, and the package size.

Notice of Privacy Practice - adequate notice of how a covered entity may use and disclose protected health information about the individual, as well as his or her rights and the covered entity's obligations with respect to that information.

NP - Nurse Practitioner.

OD - Optometrist.

Ointment - A greasy preparation, usually prepared with a petroleum jelly base, that is used to deliver medication to areas of the skin that need protection. Ointments leave oily coatings on the skin.

Omnibus Budget Reconciliation Act of 1990 (OBRA'90) - A federal law that increases pharmacists' professional responsibilities by requiring them to keep records, to perform prospective drug utilization review, and to offer to counsel patients about the proper use of their medications.

Open Panel - A network of pharmacies organized by a MCO or PBM in which all community pharmacies are invited to sign participating pharmacy agreements.

Ophthalmic Preparation - A sterile medication for the eye that may be in the form of drops or ointments.

Otic Preparation - Medication for the ear that is usually supplied in dropper bottles.

Over-the-Counter (OTC) - Medications considered to be safe to take or use without a prescription. These medications are typically stocked outside of the pharmacy department.

PA - Physician Assistant.

Parenteral - Literally means "outside of the gastrointestinal tract." Although this word is used to describe any medication given by a route of administration other than oral or rectal, it is usually used to describe injectable medications.

Parenteral (Small-Volume) - Parenteral medication that contains just enough fluid volume to safely deliver the medication into a patient's vein.

Parenteral (Large-Volume) - A parenteral medication that is used when the fluid itself is the treatment. A common example is intravenous fluids used to prevent or treat dehydration. The most complicated type of large-volume parenteral solution is total parenteral nutrition (TPN).

Participating Pharmacy Agreement - The contract between the pharmacy and the third-party payer that specifies program features such as the dispensing fee and the method of determining drug acquisition cost.

Patent - A privilege granted to an inventor that allows exclusive or sole rights to market a product or device for a limited period of time.

Patient-Controlled Analgesia (PCA) Device - A device in which pain medication is delivered at a rate determined by the patient being treated. Built-in controls prevent the patient from overdosing.

Patient Cost Sharing - The portion of a prescription expense which is paid out-of-pocket by the patient. The three most common forms of patient cost sharing are deductibles, copayments, and coinsurance.

Patient Profile - Patient record that is kept in the pharmacy department.

Pediculocide - Medication, often in the form of a shampoo, that kills lice.

Pharmacy Benefit Manager (PBM) - An organization that specializes in the management of the prescription portion of a managed health care plan. PBMs contract with participating pharmacies, process claims, control costs, and manage the various elements of the pharmacy benefit including formularies and utilization review

Point-of-Sale (POS) System - Computer technology linking pharmacies and third-party payers through telephone lines allowing eligibility verification, claims submission, claims adjudication, and utilization review at the time the prescriptions are dispensed.

Preferred Provider Organization (PPO) - A group of hospitals, physicians, and pharmacists that contracts with employers, insurance carriers, and third-party administrators to provide medical services for negotiated fees. Patients are given cost incentives (e.g., lower patient cost-sharing requirements) to use the network of "preferred providers" for services.

Prescription Container Label - Label that is affixed to the medication container that is given to the patient. These labels include patient-specific and medication-related information.

Prescription Information Label - Label that is affixed to the actual prescription order form. These labels are used to file and track prescriptions within the pharmacy department.

Prior Authorization - A requirement that specific medications be covered only if approved by the third-party payer. Usually prescribers or pharmacists have to certify that the medication is medically necessary and superior to less costly alternatives before approval is given to dispense it.

Privacy Officer - person who assures compliance with HIPAA and all other federal and state rules and regulations pertaining to the use and release of PHI.

Privacy Rule - a response to public concern over potential abuses of the privacy of health information that establishes a category of health information, referred to as protected health information, which may be used or disclosed to others in certain circumstances or under certain conditions.

PRN Refill - PRN is a Latin abbreviation that means "as needed." PRN refills for prescription medications are usually allowed for a maximum of one year.

Protected Health Information - personal, identifiable information about individuals which is created or received by a health plan, provider or health care clearinghouse.

Reconstitutable - Medication that requires the addition of distilled water or another diluent prior to dispensing and administering. Because of their short shelf lives, these medications are usually reconstituted immediately before they are dispensed.

Reconstituting Tube - A device that is used to accurately measure distilled water to be added to a medication.

Reorder Point - The minimum number of units of a particular type of merchandise that a retailer intends to keep on hand. When inventory falls to this point, it is reordered.

Reorder Quantity - The number of units that must be ordered in order to replenish the inventory to its maximum allowable level.

Returned Goods Authorization Form - A form provided by the manufacturer or wholesaler which must be completed by the pharmacy to return unused products for credit.

Rotating Stock - A method of stocking shelves in which new bottles are put at the back of the shelf and older bottles are pulled forward to help ensure that older bottles are sold first before they expire.

Schedule I (C-I) - A classification of controlled substances which includes drugs that have a high potential for abuse, no currently accepted medical use in the United States, and are unsafe for use under medical supervision. These products are not found in pharmacy departments. Examples are LSD and heroin.

Schedule II (C-II) - A classification of controlled substances which includes medications that has a currently accepted medical use in the United States and a high potential for abuse and physical or psychological dependence. Some examples are morphine (a narcotic), methamphetamine (a stimulant) and secobarbital, (a depressant).

Schedule III (C-III) - A classification of controlled substances which includes medications that have an abuse potential less than that of medications listed in Schedules I and II. Abuse of these medications may lead to moderate or low physical dependence or high psychological dependence. One example is medication with a limited quantity of narcotic medication formulated together with active non-narcotic medications (e.g., Tylenol with Codeine #3®). Certain stimulants or depressants are also included in Schedule III.

Schedule IV (C-IV) - A classification of controlled substances which includes medications that have less potential for abuse than Schedule I, II, or III medications. Abuse of these medications may lead to only a limited physical or psychological dependence. Examples include phenobarbital, Valium®, and Xanax®.

Schedule V (C-V) - A classification of controlled substances which includes medications that have limited potential for abuse and limited physical or psychological dependence. Most Schedule V medications contain limited quantities of certain narcotic medications in combination with non-narcotic active ingredients. These products are generally used as cough suppressants or as anti-diarrheals. Some examples include Novahistine® Expectorant and Lomotil®. In some states, certain Schedule V medications may be purchased in limited quantities without a prescription. However, this class of medication must be purchased at the pharmacy department and requires the patient to sign a "Schedule V Sales Record Log" and provide proof of identification.

Schedule V Sales Record Log - A type of registry which patients in some states must sign to document that they have received a Schedule V medication over-the-counter.

Shelf Life - The period during which properly stored, unopened packages of medication can be sold because their potency is still expected to be intact.

Sig - Latin abbreviation that means "you write," which is the prescriber's instructions to put the indicated directions on the prescription label.

Solution - Preparation in which the solid ingredients of medications are dissolved in a liquid (usually water).

Speed Shelf - The shelf located in the dispensing area that holds the most commonly prescribed medications.

Spirit or Essence - An alcoholic or hydroalcoholic solution. Because they contain such a high percentage of alcohol, they require storage in tight containers to prevent rapid evaporation.

Sterile - Free of bacteria or germs that can cause infection.

Stock Bottle - The original container of a drug product supplied by a manufacturer.

Subcutaneous (SubQ, SQ or SC) - Injections consisting of very small volumes of fluid (usually less than one or two milliliters) given just below the skin using a fine, short needle. Insulin and allergy shots are common examples of subcutaneous injections.

Sublingual Tablet - Tablet that dissolves rapidly when placed under the tongue and is absorbed directly into the blood stream.

Suppository - A dosage form that is usually manufactured in cylindrical, egg, or pear shapes. Some suppositories are designed for insertion into the rectum; others for insertion into the vagina.

Suspension - A preparation in which medication particles are suspended in liquid — the medication is not dissolved. To help the medication stay equally suspended, an agent is added to make the preparation thick. Suspensions must be shaken prior to use.

Surface Tension - A physical property of a liquid which causes it to cling to the sides of a container and results in the surface of the liquid to appear higher on the sides than in the middle.

Syrup - Concentrated solution of sugar in water.

Tablet - Solid dosage form that varies greatly in shape, size, weight, etc. Most tablets are swallowed whole with water and later break apart and dissolve in the digestive tract; others are designed to be chewed. Some tablets are scored so the tablet can be broken easily so patients can take a fraction of the dose.

Therapeutic Interchange - The process of selecting a drug product that is therapeutically (but not generically) equivalent to the product prescribed. To be preferred by a PBM, a therapeutic alternative is usually determined to be more cost effective than the product prescribed. Pharmacists must receive authorization from the prescribing physician in order to make a therapeutic switch.

Third-Party Prescription - A prescription that is paid, at least in part, by a private health insurance program or a government program such as Medicaid.

Third-Party Signature Log - A type of registry which patients sign to document that they have received a third-party prescription. All information entered into the log is usually found on the prescription receipt.

Total Parenteral Nutrition (TPN) - A carefully balanced solution containing sugar, protein, minerals, electrolytes, vitamins, and water administered to patients who cannot consume food or nutritional formula for a prolonged period of time.

Trade Name - Synonymous with brand name.

Transdermal Patch - A topical drug delivery system in which medication is absorbed through the skin from a patch that sticks to the skin with adhesives.

Troche or Lozenge - Tablet that is designed to be held in the mouth while it dissolves in order to keep the medication in contact with the mouth and throat for an extended period of time.

Unit-Dose System - A drug distribution system in which doses of medication are dispensed in individually packaged, ready-to-administer form.

Vaginal Tablet - A medication dosage form designed to be inserted into the vagina.

Note: See also the chapter titled "Drug and Medical Terminology".

Index

J

job description, 6
Joint Commission on Accreditation of Healthcare Organizations, 13, 62

K

Keratolytic, 230, 233 Kidney, 15, 188, 200, 210

L

laminar-flow hood, 252, 253, 257
large intestine, 208
Large-Volume Parenteral, 251, 254, 258, 260
larynx, 204, 205
Laxative, 209, 230
Leukemia, 203
Lipid, 189, 202
Liver, 15, 202, 207, 208, 209, 223, 249
long-term care facility, 43
Lot number, 144, 180, 238, 241
lotion, 59, 226
lozenge, 233
lymph node, 206, 207, 218
lymphatic and immune system, 206

M

maintenance medication, 170
Malignant, 189
Managed care, iii, 160, 161, 162, 163, 164, 165, 170
Managed indemnity, 160
manufacturer, 14, 15, 28, 33, 36, 37, 163, 168, 178, 182, 183, 241
Mark-up, 92
Mast cell stabilizer, 230
maximum allowable cost, 163, 167, 170
Medicaid, 13, 151, 162, 163, 170, 239
Medicare, 162, 163
Medicare Part D, 162
Medication allergies, 136, 139
Medication bays, 9
MedWatch, 36
Metabolism, 189, 208, 209, 215, 227, 228
Metastasis, 189
Migraine, 193, 229
Milliequivalent, 59, 90
muscular system, 200
Myocardial infarction, 203

N

Nasal congestion, 224, 233
NDC number, 33, 137, 168, 172, 179, 183, 281
needle, 86, 248, 257, 258, 259, 260
nervous system, 187, 211, 212, 228
Notice of Privacy Practice(s), 115, 119, 120, 121, 123, 124

O

Ointment, 26, 59, 94, 148, 213
Ointment jar, 26
Omnibus Budget Reconciliation Act of 1990, 13
Oncogenic, 189
Oncology, 189
open panel, 161
ophthalmic, 25
Oral contraceptive, 15, 22, 27, 148, 168, 217
Orange Book, 17, 30
Osteoarthritis, 201, 229
out-of-pocket payment, 163
Out-window, 10, 183
Ovary, 217

P

Package insert, 14, 15, 89
pancreas, 208, 209, 215
Parenteral, 17, 25, 43, 90, 168, 189, 247, 249, 250, 251
Parenteral medication, 25
Partial fill, 45, 48, 142
participating pharmacy agreement, 161, 166
patent, 28
patient controlled analgesia, 249
Patient cost sharing, 160, 163, 164, 165
Patient profile, 10, 13, 54, 114, 119, 134, 136, 140, 153
Pediatrics, 189
Penis, 218
pharmaceutical equivalence, 28
pharynx, 204, 205, 208
Pill(s), 11, 22
plunger, 257, 258
Podiatry, 189
point-of-sale, 167
Polydipsia, 189
Polyphagia, 189
Polyuria, 189
precaution, 118
Prefix, 56, 74, 187, 188
Prescription bottles, 26
Prescription container, 11, 23, 24, 140, 141, 150, 240, 241, 243
prescription information label, 140
prescription vial, 237, 239
prior authorization, 168
Privacy Officer, 121, 122, 123, 128
Privacy Rule(s), 113, 114, 115, 116, 117, 118, 119, 120, 121, 122, 123
PRN refill(s), 153
professionalism, 183
Prognosis, 188, 189
Prophylaxis, 189
proportion, 79, 80, 82, 86, 90
Protected health information, 114, 117, 119, 120, 121
Proton pump inhibitor, 61, 192, 232
pump, 61, 86, 87, 192, 200, 201, 202, 232, 260, 264
Punch cards, 237, 239

Q

Quadriplegia, 189
Quantity, 27, 44, 45, 46, 47, 48, 54, 56, 58, 61, 63, 78, 94, 95, 141, 151, 152, 154, 167, 170, 172, 178, 179, 181, 182

R

Ratio, 79, 80, 84, 86, 90
recall, 36, 37, 183
reconstitution, 146, 149
Refill, 5, 7, 8, 48, 56, 106, 107, 109, 121, 126, 132, 136, 139, 152, 153, 154, 172
reorder point, 179
reorder quantity, 179
Repackaging, iii, xiii, 17, 237, 239, 240, 241
reproductive system, 217
respiratory system, 204
returned goods authorization form, 182
Rheumatoid arthritis, 201
Roman numerals, 56, 78
Route, 25, 29, 30, 57, 60, 149, 189, 247, 248

S

Schedule I, 41, 43
Schedule II, 41, 43, 44, 45, 46, 48, 50, 153
Schedule III, 41, 43, 48, 50, 153
Schedule IV, 41, 43, 44
Schedule V, 41, 43, 46, 47, 151, 224
Schedule V Records Log, 46, 47
Schizophrenia, 194, 212
Sclerosis, 189, 212
Sepsis, 189
shelf life, 241, 250
Sign, 10, 27, 29, 44, 46, 115, 116, 151, 152, 154, 161, 180, 189
Signature log, 151, 172, 173, 184
skeletal system, 200
small intestine, 208
Small-volume parenteral, 250, 251
solution, 59, 64, 79, 80, 81, 82, 83, 86, 87, 88, 90, 233, 249, 250, 251, 255
Spasm, 189, 200
Speed shelf, 9, 181
spirit, 101
spleen, 206
state board of pharmacy, xii, 49
Sterile, iii, xiii, 11, 25, 91, 240, 247, 248, 249, 250, 251, 252, 254, 255, 256, 259, 260, 261, 262, 263, 264
Stimulant, 43, 230
Stock, 5, 7, 9, 10, 23, 24, 30, 45, 46, 48, 73, 74, 83, 93, 136, 137, 142, 144, 150, 168, 173, 177, 178, 179, 180, 181, 183, 239, 242, 264
Stock bottle, 9, 10, 23, 24, 46, 73, 74, 142, 144, 150, 168, 181, 183

Stomach, 22, 188, 208, 209, 223
Strength, 15, 29, 30, 54, 59, 74, 78, 83, 86, 103, 105, 133, 135, 137, 141, 142, 149, 153, 154, 167, 168, 181, 182, 183, 200, 230, 237, 241, 263
Stroke, 203, 212
Subcutaneous, 60, 213, 248
sublingual, 27, 28, 60
Sublingual tablet, 22
Suffix, 187, 188, 190, 191
suppository, 58, 59, 66, 230
suspension, 54, 59, 121
Symptom, 189, 230, 233
Syndrome, 189, 207, 209, 212, 218, 223, 224
syringe, 86, 257, 258, 259
syrup, 22, 59, 81
ystolic blood pressure, 203

T

Tablet, 21, 34, 54, 56, 58, 59, 66, 74, 94, 181, 217, 243
Tachycardia, 203
Therapeutic interchange, 30, 170
Third party, 118, 135
Third-party prescription, 151, 153, 166, 168
third-party program, 134, 138, 151, 159, 160, 168, 174
Tinea pedis, 214
trachea, 204
trade name, 28
Traditional indemnity, 160
Transdermal patch, 25
Transfer, 45, 48, 49, 108, 109, 149, 179, 189, 256
Transfer warning statement, 49
tubing, 254, 260, 261, 264

U

Unit-dose, 237, 238, 239
ureter, 210
Urethra, 210, 211, 218
urinary system, 210
Uterus, 217, 218

V

Vagina, 25, 218
Vaginal tablet, 25
vertical laminar-flow hood, 253
voluntary, 36, 162, 200, 211

W

warehouse, 177, 182
Warning, 28, 49, 117, 121, 149
Wart, 25, 214, 226
wholesaler, 36, 37, 177, 179, 180, 182
Word root, 187, 188

Appendix
Most Frequently Prescribed Medications

Note: These are the top 200 drugs by NDC number; therefore, some drugs are listed several times. This is because several companies often manufacture products with the same generic name. If you would like this list sorted by generic name or by indication, or for any updates to *The National Pharmacy Technician Training Program, 6th Edition*, please visit http://www.nationaltechexam.org/

Rank	Product (Brand/generic)	(Generic name)	Most common use(s)	Therapeutic Class
1	hydrocodone, acetaminophen (e.g. Lorcet, Lortab, Norco, Vicodin)	(hydrocodone and acetaminophen)	Pain treatment	Narcotic analgesic
2	lisinopril (e.g. Prinivil, Zestril)	(lisinopril)	High blood pressure or heart failure treatment	ACE-Inhibitor (ACE-I)
3	Lipitor	(atorvastatin)	High cholesterol treatment	HMG-CoA reductase inhibitor
4	Amoxil, Trimox	(amoxicillin)	Bacterial infection treatment	Penicillin
5	Levothyroxine	(levothyroxine sodium)	Thyroid hormone deficiency treatment	Thyroid hormone replacement
6	hydroclorothiazide	(hydrochlorothiazide)	High blood pressure treatment	Diuretic
7	azithromycin (e.g. Zithromax, Zithromax Z-Pak)	(azithromycin)	Bacterial infection treatment	Macrolide
8	atenolol (e.g. Tenormin)	(atenolol)	High blood pressure or chest pain treatment	Beta-blocker
9	simvastatin (e.g. Zocor)	(simvastatin)	High cholesterol treatment	HMG-CoA reductase inhibitor
10	alprazolam (e.g. Xanax)	(alprazolam)	Anxiety treatment	Benzodiazepine
11	furosemide (e.g. Lasix)	(furosemide)	Edema or hypertension treatment	Loop diuretic
12	metformin (e.g. Glucophage)	(metformin HCl)	Glycemic control improvement	Biguanide
13	sertraline (e.g. Zoloft)	(sertraline HCl)	Depression or anxiety treatment	Selective serotonin receptor inhibitor
14	metoprolol tartrate (e.g. Lopressor)	(metoprolol Tart)	High blood pressure treatment	Beta-blocker
15	Singulair	(montelukast)	Asthma and/or allergies treatment/ prevention	Leukotriene receptor antagonist
16	Lexapro	(escitalopram)	Depression or anxiety treatment	Selective serotonin reuptake inhibitor
17	Nexium	(esomeprazole)	Ulcers or reflux (GERD) treatment	Proton pump inhibitor
18	Synthroid	(Levothyroxine sodium)	Thyroid hormone deficiency treatment	Thyroid hormone replacement
19	ibuprofen (e.g. Motrin)	(ibuprofen Rx)	Pain treatment	NSAID
20	amlodipine besylate (e.g. Norvasc)	(amlodipine besylate)	High blood pressure treatment	Calcium channel blocker (CCB)
21	oxycodone, acetaminophen (e.g. Percocet, Tylox, Roxicet, Endocet)	(oxycodone and acetaminophen)	Pain treatment	Narcotic analgesic
22	Prednisone	(prednisone)	Treat variety of diseases including, but not limited to: acute allergy, inflammation, asthma organ transplantation.	Oral corticosteroid
23	cephalexin	(cephalexin)	Bacterial infection treatment	Cephalosporin (1st generation)
24	fluoxetine (e.g. Prozac)	(fluoxetine HCl)	Depression or anxiety treatment	Selective serotonin receptor inhibitor
25	Plavix	(clopidogrel)	Blood clot prevention	Antiplatelet agent
26	triamterene with hydroclorothiazine (e.g. Dyazide, Maxzide)	(triamterene and hydrochlorothiazide)	High blood pressure treatment	Combination thiazide and potassium-sparing diuretic
27	Toprol-XL	(metroprolol-XL)	High blood pressure, heart failure, or chest pain treatment	Beta-blocker

Rank	Product (Brand/generic)	(Generic name)	Most common use(s)	Therapeutic Class
28	propoxyphene and acetaminophen (e.g. Darvocet)	(propoxyphene and acetaminophen)	Pain treatment	Narcotic analgesic
29	warfarin	(warfarin sodium)	Blood clot prevention	Anticoagulant
30	lorazepam (e.g. Ativan)	(lorazepam)	Anxiety treatment	Benzodiazepine
31	omeprazole (e.g. Prilosec)	(omeprazole)	Ulcers or reflux (GERD) treatment	Proton pump inhibitor
32	Prevacid	(lansoprazole)	Ulcers or reflux (GERD) treatment	Proton pump inhibitor
33	clonazepam (e.g. Klonopin)	(clonazepam)	Anxiety treatment	Benzodiazepine
34	amoxicillin and clavulanate (e.g. Augmentin)	(amoxicillin and clavulanate)	Bacterial infection treatment	Penicillin
35	Vytorin	(simvastatin and ezetimibe)	High cholesterol treatment	Combination HMG-CoA reductase inhibitor and 2-azetidinone
36	albuterol aerosol	(albuterol)	Asthma treatment	Beta2-agonist
37	ciprofloxacin (e.g. Cipro)	(ciprofloxacin HCl)	Bacterial infection treatment	Quinolone
38	metoprolol succinate	(metoprolol succinate)	High blood pressure treatment	Beta-blocker
39	cyclobenzaprine (e.g. Flexeril)	(cyclobenzaprine)	Muscle spasm pain treatment	Skeletal muscle relaxant
40	tramadol (e.g. Ultram)	(tramadol)	Pain treatment	Non-narcotic analgesic
41	Advair Diskus	(fluticasone and salmeterol)	Asthma treatment/prevention	Combination oral corticosteroid and long-acting beta2-agonist
42	gabapentin (e.g. Neurotin)	(gabapentin)	Seizures control, postherpetic neuralgia management	Anticonvulsant
43	Zyrtec	(cetirizine)	Allergy treatment/ prevention	Antihistamine
44	fexofenadine (e.g. Allegra)	(fexofenadine HCl)	Allergy treatment/ prevention	Antihistamine
45	Effexor XR	(venlafaxine)	Depression or anxiety treatment	Serotonin/Norephinephrine reuptake inhibitor
46	lisinopril, hydrochlorothiazide (e.g. Prinzide, Zestoretic)	(lisinopril and hydrochlorothiazide)	High blood pressure or heart failure treatment	Combination ACE-I and diuretic
47	citalopram (e.g. Celexa)	(citalopram)	Depression or anxiety treatment	Selective serotonin receptor inhibitor
48	Protonix	(pantoprazole)	Ulcers or reflux (GERD) treatment	Proton pump inhibitor
49	paroxetine HCl (e.g. Paxil)	(paroxetine HCl)	Depression or anxiety treatment	Selective serotonin receptor inhibitor
50	trazodone HCl (e.g. Desyrel)	(trazodone HCl)	Depression treatment	Serotonin reuptake inhibitor
51	lovastatin (e.g. Mevacor)	(lovastatin)	High cholesterol treatment	HMG-CoA reductase inhibitor
52	Diovan	(valsartan)	High blood pressure or heart failure treatment	Angiotensin receptor blocker (ARB)
53	Fosamax	(alendronate)	Osteoporosis treatment and prevention	Bisphosphonate
54	clonidine (e.g. Catapres)	(clonidine HCl)	High blood pressure treatment	Alpha2-agonist
55	fluticasone (e.g. Flonase)	(fluticasone)	Asthma and/or allergies treatment/ prevention	Nasal corticosteroid
56	zolpidem tartrate	(zolpidem tartrate)	Insomnia treatment	Hypnotic
57	Zetia	(ezetimibe)	High cholesterol treatment	2-Azetidinone

Rank	Product (Brand/generic)	(Generic name)	Most common use(s)	Therapeutic Class
58	acetaminophen with codeine (e.g. Tylenol with Codeine)	(acetaminophen and codeine)	Pain treatment	Narcotic analgesic
59	Crestor	(rosuvastatin)	High cholesterol treatment	HMG-CoA reductase inhibitor
60	potassium chloride	(potassium chloride)	Potassium deficiency treatment	Electrolyte supplement
61	Levaquin	(levofloxacin)	Bacterial infection treatment	Quinolone
62	amitriptyline (e.g. Elavil)	(amitriptyline)	Depression treatment	Tricyclic antidepressant
63	diazepam (e.g. Valium)	(diazepam)	Anxiety treatment	Benzodiazepine
64	naproxen (e.g. Naprosyn)	(naproxen)	Pain treatment	NSAID
65	enalapril (e.g. Vasotec)	(enalapril)	High blood pressure or heart failure treatment	ACE-Inhibitor (ACE-I)
66	Diovan HCT	(valsartan and hydrochlorothiazide)	High blood pressure treatment	Combination ARB and diuretic
67	Klor-Con	(potassium chloride)	Potassium deficiency treatment	Electrolyte supplement
68	ranitidine HCl (e.g. Zantac)	(ranitidine HCl)	Ulcers or reflux (GERD) treatment	H2-antagonist
69	Cymbalta	(duloxetine)	Depression or diabetic neuropathic pain treatment	Serotonin/Norephinephrine reuptake inhibitor
70	fluconazole (e.g. Diflucan)	(fluconazole)	Fungal infection treatment	Antifungal
71	Actos	(pioglitazone)	Glycemic control improvement	Thiazolidinedione
72	carisoprodol	(carisoprodol)	Muscle spasm pain treatment	Muscle relaxant
73	Premarin	(conjugated estrogens)	Menopausal symptom treatment	Estrogen derivative
74	allopurinol (e.g. Zyloprim)	(allopurinol)	Gout (high uric acid levels) prevention	Xanthine Oxidase Inhibitor
75	ProAir HFA	(albuterol sulfate)	Asthma, chronic bronchitis	Bronchodilator
76	doxycycline hyclate (e.g. Vibramycin)	(doxycycline hyclate)	Bacterial infection treatment	Tetracycline
77	Celebrex	(celecoxib)	Pain, inflammation	COX-2 inhibitor
78	methylprednisolone	(methylprednisolone)	Pain, inflammation	Corticosteroid
79	Flomax	(tamsulosin)	Prostate / urinary disorder treatment	Alpha1-blocker
80	Seroquel	(quetiapine)	Schizophrenia treatment	Antipsychotic (Atypical)
81	clonidine	(clonidine HCl)	High blood pressure treatment	Alpha 2 agonist
82	Norvasc	(amlodipine besylate)	High blood pressure treatment	Calcium channel blocker (CCB)
83	Nasonex	(mometasone)	Allergy treatment/ prevention	Corticosteroid
84	sulfamethaxazole and trimethoprim (e.g. Bactrim, Septra)	(sulfamethaxazole and trimethoprim)	Bacterial infection treatment	Combination sulfonamide and trimethoprim
85	promethazine (e.g. Phenergan)	(promethazine)	Nausea control	Antiemetic
86	Tricor	(fenofibrate)	High cholesterol treatment	Cholesterol lowering agent
87	Lantus	(insulin glargine)	Glycemic control improvement	Insulin
88	Viagra	(sildenafil)	Erectile dysfunction treatment	Phosphodiesterase-5 inhibitor
89	isosorbide mononitrate (e.g. Imdur)	(isosorbide mononitrate)	Chest pain prevention	Vasodilator
90	Altace	(ramipril)	High blood pressure or heart failure treatment	ACE-Inhibitor (ACE-I)
91	Yasmin	(drospirenone and ethinyl estradiol)	Pregnancy prevention	Oral contraceptive

Rank	Product (Brand/generic)	(Generic name)	Most common use(s)	Therapeutic Class
92	pravastatin (e.g. Pravachol)	(pravastatin)	High cholesterol treatment	HMG-CoA reductase inhibitor
93	Levoxyl	(levothyroxine sodium)	Thyroid hormone deficiency treatment	Thyroid hormone replacement
94	Adderall XR	(amphetamine and dextroamphetamine)	Attention deficit hyperactivity disorder (ADHD) control	Stimulant
95	meloxicam (e.g. Mobic)	(meloxicam)	Arthritis treatment	NSAID
96	Lotrel	(benazepril and amlodipine)	High blood pressure treatment	Combination ACE-I and CCB
97	Actonel	(risedronate)	Osteoporosis treatment and prevention	Bisphosphonate
98	Ambien CR	(zolpidem)	Insomnia treatment	Hypnotic
99	verapamil SR (e.g. Calan SR, Verelan PM)	(verapamil SR)	High blood pressure, chest pain, or irregular heartbeat treatment	Calcium Channel Blocker (CCB)
100	Cozaar	(losartan)	High blood pressure or heart failure treatment	Angiotensin receptor blocker (ARB)
101	folic acid	(folic acid)	Anemia (folic acid deficiency) treatment and prevention	Vitamin
102	Coreg	(carvedilol)	High blood pressure or heart failure treatment	Beta-blocker
103	glyburide (e.g. Diabeta)	(glyburide)	Glycemic control improvement	Sulfonylurea
104	penicillin VK (e.g. Veetids)	(penicillin VK)	Bacterial infection treatment	Penicillin
105	spironolactone (e.g. Aldactone)	(spironolactone)	Edema or hypertension treatment	Diuretic
106	Valtrex	(valaciclovir)	Viral infection treatment	Antiviral
107	Lyrica	(pregabalin)	Diabetic neuropathic pain treatment	Gamma Aminobutyric Acid
108	temazepam (e.g. Restoril)	(temazepam)	Anxiety or insomnia treatment	Antianxiety, hypnotic
109	Concerta	(methylphenidate)	Attention deficit hyperactivity disorder (ADHD) control	Stimulant
110	glimepiride (e.g. Amaryl)	(glimepiride)	Type 2 diabetes mellitus	Anti-diabetic
111	Ambien	(zolpidem)	Insomnia treatment	Hypnotic
112	Risperdal	(risperidone)	Schizophrenia treatment	Antipsychotic (Atypical)
113	albuterol neb solution	(albuterol neb solution)	Asthma, chronic bronchitis	Bronchodilator
114	Digitek	(digoxin)	Heart failure or irregular heartbeat treatment	Cardiac glycoside
115	Topamax	(topiramate)	Seizure control	Anticonvulsant
116	triamcinolone acet topical	(triamcinolone acet topical)	Skin inflammation and irritation	Topical steroid
117	Chantix	(varenicline)	Smoking cessation	Nicotine receptor agonist
118	clindamycin	(clindamycin)	Infections	Antibiotic
119	Avandia	(rosiglitazone)	Glycemic control improvement	Thiazolidinedione
120	metformin HCl ER	(metformin HCl ER)	Type 2 diabetes mellitus	Anti-diabetic
121	Lamictal	(lamotrigine)	Seizure control	Anticonvulsant
122	Ortho-Tri-Cyclen Lo	(norgestimate and ethinyl estradiol)	Pregnancy prevention	Oral contraceptive
123	glipizide	(glipizide)	Glycemic control improvement	Sulfonylurea
124	benazepril	(benazepril)	High blood pressure treatment	ACE-Inhibitor (ACE-I)

284

Rank	Product (Brand/generic)	(Generic name)	Most common use(s)	Therapeutic Class
125	Xalatan	(latanoprost)	Glaucoma treatment	Antiglaucoma (Prostaglandin Analog)
126	Aciphex	(rabeprazole)	Ulcers or reflux (GERD) treatment	Proton pump inhibitor
127	metronidazole (e.g. Flagyl)	(metronidazole)	Infections	Anti-bacterial
128	Hyzaar	(losartan and hydrochlorothiazide)	High blood pressure treatment	Combination ARB and diuretic
129	Spiriva Handihaler	(tiotropium)	Bronchitis, emphysema COPD treatment	Anticholinergic
130	Wellbutrin XL	(bupropion)	Depression treatment	Dopamine-reuptake inhibitor
131	metoclopramide (e.g. Reglan)	(metoclopramide)	Heart burn, stomach problems	Dopamin receptor antagonist
132	Lunesta	(eszopiclone)	Insomnia treatment	Hypnotic
133	quinapril (e.g. Accupril)	(quinapril)	High blood pressure or heart failure treatment	ACE-inhibitor (ACE-I)
134	Benicar	(olmesartan)	High blood pressure or heart failure treatment	Angiotensin receptor blocker (ARB)
135	glipizide ER (e.g. Glucotrol XL)	(glipizide ER)	Glycemic control improvement	Sulfonylurea
136	propranolol HCl	(propranolol HCl)	High blood pressure treatment	Beta-blocker
137	hydroxyzine (e.g. Atarax, Vistaril)	(hydroxyzine)	Relief of itching and allergic skin reactions, nausea/vomiting	Antihistamine
138	Benicar HCT	(olmesartan and hydrochlorothiazide)	High blood pressure treatment	Combination ARB and diuretic
139	Aricept	(donepezil)	Alzheimers-type dementia treatment	Acetylcholinesterase inhibitor
140	diclofenac sodium	(diclofenac sodium)	Pain, inflammation	NSAID
141	Avapro	(irbesartan)	High blood pressure or heart failure treatment	Angiotensin receptor blocker (ARB)
142	estradiol oral	(estradiol oral)	Menopausal symptom treatment	Hormone
143	gemfibrozil	(gemfibrozil)	High cholesterol treatment	Fibrate anticholesterolemic
144	Detrol LA	(tolterodine)	Urinary control improvement	Antispasmotic, anticholinergic
145	oxycodone ER	(oxycodone)	Pain treatment	Narcotic analgesic
146	doxazosin (e.g. Cardura)	(doxazosin)	High blood pressure	Alpha blocker
147	meclizine	(meclizine)	Motion sickness treatment and prevention	Antihistamine
148	Trinessa-28	(ethinyl estradiol/norgestimate)	Pregnancy prevention	Oral contraceptive
149	Cialis	(tadalafil)	Erectile dysfunction treatment	Phosphodiesterase-5 inhibitor
150	Combivent	(albuterol and ipratropium)	Asthma treatment	Combination beta2-agonist and anticholinergic agent
151	mirtazapine	(mirtazapine)	Depression, anxiety	Anti-depressant
152	nitrofurantoin monohydrate	(nitrofurantoin monohydrate)	Urinary tract infections	Antibiotic
153	glyburide/metformin HCl	(glyburide/metformin HCl)	Type 2 diabetes mellitus	Anti-diabetic
154	Budeprion XL	(buproprion extended release)	Depression	Anti-depressant
155	Acyclovir	(acyclovir)	Viral infection treatment	Antiviral

Rank	Product (Brand/generic)	(Generic name)	Most common use(s)	Therapeutic Class
156	amphetamine salt comb	(amphetamine Salt comb)	Attention deficit hyperactivity disorder (ADHD) control	Stimulant
157	Yaz	(drospirenone and ethinyl estradiol)	Pregnancy prevention	Oral contraceptive
158	Glycolax	(polyethylene glycol)	Constipation treatment	Laxative
159	Imitrex	(sumatriptan)	Migraine treatment	Serotonin 5-HT agonist
160	Evista	(raloxifene)	Osteoporosis treatment and prevention	Bisphosphonate
161	NuvaRing	(etonogestrel and ethinyl estradiol)	Pregnancy prevention	Contraceptive
162	Cartia XT	(diltiazem XT)	High blood pressure, chest pain, or irregular heartbeat treatment	Calcium Channel Blocker (CCB)
163	Omnicef	(cefdinir)	Bacterial infection treatment	Cephalosporin (3rd generation)
164	Niaspan	(niacin)	High cholesterol treatment	Misc. cholesterol lowering agent
165	fentanyl transdermal (e.g. Duragesic)	(fentanyl transfermal)	Chronic pain	Opioid narcotic
166	buspirone HCl (e.g. BuSpar)	(buspirone HCl)	Anxiety	Anti-anxiety
167	Tri-Sprintec-28	(norgestimate and ethinyl estradiol)	Pregnancy prevention	Oral contraceptive
168	nabumetone (e.g. Relafen)	(nabumetone)	Pain and inflammation	NSAID
169	Diltiazem CD	(diltiazem CD)	High blood pressure treatment	Calcium Channel Blocker (CCB)
170	Boniva	(ibandronate)	Osteoporosis treatment and prevention	Biphosphonate
171	promethazine/codeine	(promethazine/codeine)	Nausea control	Antiemetic
172	methotrexate	(methotrexate)	Cancer, rheumatoid arthritis	Antimetabolite
173	bisoprolol/HCTZ	(bisoprolol/HCTZ)	High blood pressure treatment	Beta-blocker
174	oxycodone	(oxycodone)	Pain	Narcotic analgesic
175	Flovent HFA	(fluticasone)	Asthma and/or allergies treatment/ prevention	Nasal corticosteroid
176	butalbital/APAP/caffeine	(butalbital/APAP/caffeine)	Pain treatment	Analgesic
177	phentermine	(phentermine)	Weight loss	Stimulant
178	Avelox	(moxifloxacin)	Bacterial infection treatment	Antibiotic
179	clotrimazole/betamethasone	(clotrimazole/betamethasone)	Ringworm, tinea infections	Corticosteroid/antifungal
180	minocycline	(minocycline)	Infections	Antibiotic
181	Abilify	(aripiprazole)	Schizophrenia treatment	Antipsychotic (Atypical)
182	Avalide	(irbesartan and hydrochlorothiazide)	High blood pressure treatment	Combination ARB and thiazide diuretic
183	Nifedipine ER	(nifedipine ER)	High blood pressure, chest pain, or irregular heartbeat treatment	Calcium Channel Blocker (CCB)
184	cefdinir	(cefdinir)	Infections	Cephalosporin antibiotic
185	terazosin	(terazosin)	High blood pressure	Alpha-1 antagonist
186	bupropion SR (e.g. Wellbutrin)	(bupropion SR)	Depression	Anti-depressant
187	Requip	(ropinirole)	Parkinson's disease	Anti-Parkinson

Rank	Product (Brand/generic)	(Generic name)	Most common use(s)	Therapeutic Class
188	Zyrtec Syrup	(cetirizine)	Allergy treatment/ prevention	Antihistamine
189	Coumadin	(warfarin Sodium)	Blood clot prevention	Anticoagulant
190	Zyprexa	(olanzapine)	Schizophrenia treatment	Antipsychotic (Atypical)
191	Depakote ER	(divalproex)	Seizure control	Anticonvulsant
192	Mupirocin	(mupirocin)	Skin infections	Antibiotic
193	Nasacort AQ	(triamcinolone)	Allergy treatment/ prevention	Nasal corticosteroid
194	felodipine ER	(felodipine ER)	High blood pressure, chest pain, or irregular heartbeat treatment	Calcium Channel Blocker (CCB)
195	potassium chloride	(potassium chloride E)	Potassium deficiency treatment	Electrolyte supplement
196	tramadol HCl/APAP	(Tramadol HCl/APAP)	Pain	Analgesic
197	Skelaxin	(metaxalone)	Pain and muscle stiffness	Muscle relaxant
198	tizanidine HCl	(tizanidine HCl)	Muscle spasm pain treatment	Muscle relaxant
199	ferrous sulfate	(ferrous sulfate)	Iron deficiency	Vitamin/Mineral
200	Allegra-D 12 hour	(fexofenadine and pseudoephedrine)	Allergy treatment/ prevention	Antihistamine

Source: Top 200 Brand Drugs by units in 2007. Drug Topics Feb 25, 2008.
http://drugtopics.modernmedicine.com/drugtopics/data/articlestandard//drugtopics/072008/491207/article.pdf Accessed April 20, 2008

Exam for the Certification of Pharmacy Technicians

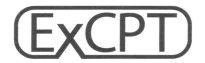

$54.0
ISBN 978-0-615-21118-
5540

9 780615 211183

"The Exceptional Alternative for Pharmacy Technician Certification"

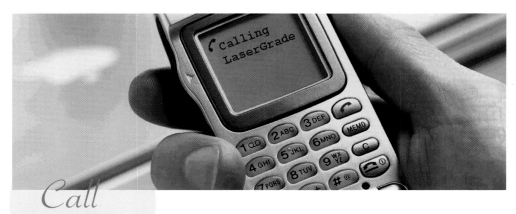

Call

LaserGrade at **800.211.2754** to arrange a test date, time and location that best fits your schedule.

A nationally recognized and psychometrically sound pharmacy technician certification exam. For more information, visit www.nationaltechexam.org

2536 S. Old Highway 94, Suite 214 • St. Charles, MO 63303 • *office:* 314.442.6775 • *toll free tech line:* 866.391.9188

ExCPT *Exam Details*

- Proctored computer-based exam consists of 110 multiple-choice items

- Candidates are given 2 hours to take the exam

- Psychometrically sound and applicable to all pharmacy practice sites

- Diagnostic report provided immediately to unsuccessful candidates

www.nationaltechexam.org

Less Expensive

The ExCPT Exam is the most economical pharmacy technician test available today. Cost can be found at our website www.nationaltechexam.org.

More Convenient

The ExCPT Exam is offered in over 600 LaserGrade Testing Centers located throughout the U.S. You can schedule and take the exam almost any time you like.

Immediate Results

The ExCPT Exam provides reports to candidates Immediately after the exam. There is no need to wait 6–8 weeks for results.